The Big List of low sodium foods

Keep your daily sodium intake low

D1519360

Copyrights

No part of the materials available through this book (except for personal use) may be copied, photocopied, reproduced, translated or reduced to any electronic medium or machine-readable form, in whole or in part, without prior written consent of the publisher.

Disclaimer

The information contained in this book should be used aa a reference only, and it is not intended to give any medical advice.

Forward

Food choices is important to lower the daily sodium intake, more than 40%of the sodium consumed by Americans is coming from fast foods, pop corns, and egg dishes...

Too much sodium can cause severe health problems like high blood pressure, heart diseases, and strokes...

As recommended by the **U.S. Food and Drug Administration,** the daily intake of sodium to stay in a good health should not exceed **2300 mg per day, or a %DV that is less than 100%.**

%DV: as defined by USDA, the %DV is is the percentage of the Daily Value for each nutrient in a serving of the food and shows how much of a nutrient contributes to a total daily diet.

You can use either the sodium content in mg, or the %DV to verify the sodium content in a food in this list. (See more explanation in the "How to use this list" section).

When you buy canned foods, always look at the label to see the sodium content or **the sodium %DV** of the food. See example in the next page:

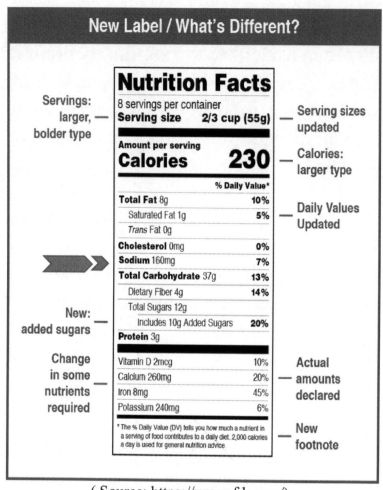

(Source: https://www.fda.gov/)

From the above picture, the %DV of the sodium is 7%, which still less than 100%.

How to use this list

1. The list is organized by alphabet from A to Z, so in order to find out if a food is low in sodium or not, just look for it in this list as you would normally do if you use a dictionary, then look at the letter in the left column:

   - **L**: Stands for "**low in sodium**"
   - **M**: Stands for "**Medium in sodium**"
   - **H**: Stands for "**high in sodium**"
   - **V.H**: Stands for "**Very high in sodium**"

2. Sometimes you need to look for the food category to find the food you are looking for, for example: you may not find "peanut bar" in the foods that

start by letter "P", but when you search in the category of Candies, then you will find it, same for Oats for example, you will find it in the "Cereals" food category…

3. When you want to buy canned foods, then use the last two columns in this list to choose foods that have %DV less than 7%

	Food	Sodium content (in mg)	%DV
L	Acerola juice, raw,	0	0%
L	Alcoholic beer,	0	0%
L	Almond milk, chocolate, ready-to-drink,	71	3%
L	Almond milk, sweetened, vanilla flavor, ready-to-drink,	63	3%
L	Almond milk, unsweetened, shelf stable,	71	3%
L	Amaranth grain, uncooked,	0	0%

	Food	Sodium content (in mg)	%DV
L	Acerola juice, raw,	0	0%
L	Alcoholic beer,	0	0%
L	Almond milk, chocolate, ready-to-drink,	71	3%
L	Almond milk, sweetened, vanilla flavor, ready-to-drink,	63	3%
L	Almond milk, unsweetened, shelf stable,	71	3%
L	Amaranth grain, uncooked,	0	0%
M	Amaranth leaves, cooked, boiled, drained, with salt,	257	11%
L	Apple juice, canned or bottled, unsweetened	0	0%
L	Apples, raw, with skin,	0	0%
L	Apples, raw, without skin,	0	0%
L	Applesauce, canned, sweetened, without salt	0	0%
L	Apricot nectar, canned,	0	0%
L	Apricot nectar, canned, without added ascorbic acid,	0	0%
L	Apricots, dried, sulfured, stewed, without added sugar,	0	0%
L	Apricots, frozen, sweetened,	0	0%
L	Apricots, raw,	0	0%
M	Arrowhead, cooked, boiled, drained, with salt,	254	11%
L	Arrowroot flour,	0	0%
M	Artichokes, (globe or french), cooked, boiled, drained, with salt,	296	13%
L	Artichokes, (globe or french), cooked, boiled, drained, without salt,	60	3%
M	Asparagus, canned, drained solids,	287	12%
M	Asparagus, canned, regular pack, solids and liquids,	284	12%
M	Asparagus, cooked, boiled, drained, with salt,	240	10%
L	Asparagus, raw,	0	0%
L	Avocados, raw, florida,	0	0%
L	Babyfood, apple-banana juice,	0	0%
L	Babyfood, apple-cranberry juice,	0	0%
L	Babyfood, cereal, high protein, prepared with whole milk,	49	2%

L	Babyfood, cereal, high protein, with apple and orange, dry,	104	5%
L	Babyfood, cereal, high protein, with apple and orange, prepared with whole milk,	58	3%
L	Babyfood, cereal, mixed, dry fortified,	0	0%
L	Babyfood, cereal, mixed, prepared with whole milk,	42	2%
L	Babyfood, cereal, mixed, with applesauce and bananas, junior, fortified,	0	0%
L	Babyfood, cereal, mixed, with applesauce and bananas, strained,	0	0%
L	Babyfood, cereal, mixed, with bananas, dry,	0	0%
L	Babyfood, cereal, mixed, with bananas, prepared with whole milk,	48	2%
L	Babyfood, cereal, mixed, with honey, prepared with whole milk,	48	2%
L	Babyfood, cereal, oatmeal, prepared with whole milk,	46	2%
L	Babyfood, cereal, oatmeal, with applesauce and bananas, junior, fortified,	0	0%
L	Babyfood, cereal, oatmeal, with applesauce and bananas, strained,	0	0%
L	Babyfood, cereal, oatmeal, with bananas, prepared with whole milk,	48	2%
L	Babyfood, cereal, oatmeal, with honey, dry,	47	2%
L	Babyfood, cereal, oatmeal, with honey, prepared with whole milk,	49	2%
L	Babyfood, cereal, rice with pears and apple, dry, instant fortified,	0	0%
L	Babyfood, cereal, rice, prepared with whole milk,	42	2%
L	Babyfood, cereal, rice, with applesauce and bananas, strained,	0	0%
L	Babyfood, cereal, rice, with bananas, dry,	0	0%
L	Babyfood, cereal, rice, with bananas, prepared with whole milk,	47	2%
L	Babyfood, cereal, rice, with honey, prepared with whole milk,	49	2%
L	Babyfood, cereal, with eggs, strained,	38	2%
L	Babyfood, cherry cobbler, junior,	0	0%

M	Babyfood, cookies,	300	13%
L	Babyfood, green beans, dices, toddler,	37	2%
L	Babyfood, juice treats, fruit medley, toddler,	89	4%
L	Babyfood, juice, apple - cherry,	0	0%
L	Babyfood, juice, apple and cherry,	0	0%
L	Babyfood, juice, apple and grape,	0	0%
L	Babyfood, juice, apple and peach,	0	0%
L	Babyfood, juice, apple and plum,	0	0%
L	Babyfood, juice, apple-sweet potato,	0	0%
L	Babyfood, juice, apple, with calcium,	0	0%
L	Babyfood, juice, fruit punch, with calcium,	0	0%
L	Babyfood, juice, orange and apple and banana,	0	0%
L	Babyfood, juice, orange and apple,	0	0%
L	Babyfood, juice, orange and banana,	0	0%
L	Babyfood, juice, orange and pineapple,	0	0%
L	Babyfood, juice, orange,	0	0%
L	Babyfood, juice, prune and orange,	0	0%
L	Babyfood, macaroni and cheese, toddler,	112	5%
M	Babyfood, mashed cheddar potatoes and broccoli, toddlers,	176	8%
M	Bagels, cinnamon-raisin,	344	15%
M	Bagels, cinnamon-raisin, toasted,	370	16%
H	Bagels, egg,	505	22%
M	Bagels, multigrain,	359	16%
H	Bagels, oat bran,	590	26%
M	Bagels, plain, enriched, with calcium propionate (includes onion, poppy, sesame),	422	18%
M	Bagels, plain, enriched, with calcium propionate (includes onion, poppy, sesame), toasted,	457	20%
H	Bagels, plain, enriched, without calcium propionate (includes onion, poppy, sesame),	534	23%
H	Bagels, plain, unenriched, with calcium propionate (includes onion, poppy, sesame),	534	23%
H	Bagels, plain, unenriched, without calcium propionate(includes onion, poppy, sesame),	534	23%
M	Bagels, wheat,	439	19%
M	Bagels, whole grain white,	372	16%

L	Baking chocolate, mexican, squares,	0	0%
M	Balsam-pear (bitter gourd), leafy tips, cooked, boiled, drained, with salt,	249	11%
M	Balsam-pear (bitter gourd), pods, cooked, boiled, drained, with salt,	242	11%
L	Balsam-pear (bitter gourd), pods, raw,	0	0%
M	Bamboo shoots, cooked, boiled, drained, with salt,	240	10%
L	Bamboo shoots, raw,	0	0%
L	Bamboo shoots, raw, cooked, boiled, drained, without salt,	0	0%
L	Bananas, dehydrated, or banana powder,	0	0%
L	Bananas, raw,	0	0%
L	Barley flour or meal,	0	0%
L	Barley, pearled, cooked,	0	0%
L	Basil, fresh,	0	0%
M	Beans, adzuki, mature seed, cooked, boiled, with salt,	244	11%
M	Beans, adzuki, mature seeds, canned, sweetened,	218	9%
L	Beans, adzuki, mature seeds, raw,	0	0%
L	Beans, baked, canned, no salt added,	0	0%
M	Beans, baked, canned, plain or vegetarian,	343	15%
H	Beans, baked, canned, with beef,	475	21%
M	Beans, baked, canned, with franks,	430	19%
M	Beans, baked, home prepared,	422	18%
M	Beans, black turtle, mature seeds, canned,	384	17%
M	Beans, black turtle, mature seeds, cooked, boiled, with salt,	239	10%
L	Beans, black turtle, mature seeds, cooked, boiled, without salt,	0	0%
M	Beans, black, mature seeds, canned, low sodium,	138	6%
M	Beans, black, mature seeds, cooked, boiled, with salt,	237	10%
L	Beans, black, mature seeds, cooked, boiled, without salt,	0	0%
L	Beans, black, mature seeds, raw,	0	0%
M	Beans, kidney, all types, mature seeds, canned,	296	13%

M	Beans, kidney, all types, mature seeds, cooked, boiled, with salt,	238	10%
L	Beans, kidney, all types, mature seeds, cooked, boiled, without salt,	0	0%
L	Beans, mung, mature seeds, sprouted, canned, drained solids,	42	2%
M	Beans, navy, mature seeds, canned,	336	15%
M	Beans, navy, mature seeds, cooked, boiled, with salt,	237	10%
L	Beans, navy, mature seeds, cooked, boiled, without salt,	0	0%
M	Beans, snap, yellow, cooked, boiled, drained, with salt,	239	10%
L	Beans, snap, yellow, cooked, boiled, drained, without salt,	0	0%
L	Beef composite, separable lean only, trimmed to 1\8\ fat, choice, cooked,	53	2%
M	Beef macaroni with tomato sauce, frozen entree, reduced fat,	178	8%
M	Beef pot pie, frozen entree, prepared,	365	16%
H	Beef sausage, fresh, cooked,	813	35%
H	Beef sausage, pre-cooked,	822	36%
M	Beef stew, canned entree,	388	17%
H	Beef, bologna, reduced sodium,	682	30%
L	Beef, brisket, whole, separable lean only, all grades, raw,	79	3%
L	Beef, carcass, separable lean and fat, choice, raw,	59	3%
L	Beef, carcass, separable lean and fat, select, raw,	59	3%
L	Beef, grass-fed, ground, raw,	68	3%
L	Beef, grass-fed, strip steaks, lean only, raw,	55	2%
M	Beef, variety meats and by-products, brain, cooked, pan-fried,	158	7%
L	Beef, variety meats and by-products, brain, cooked, simmered,	108	5%
L	Beef, variety meats and by-products, brain, raw,	126	5%
L	Beef, variety meats and by-products, heart, cooked, simmered,	59	3%

L	Beef, variety meats and by-products, heart, raw,	98	4%
L	Beef, variety meats and by-products, kidneys, cooked, simmered,	94	4%
M	Beef, variety meats and by-products, kidneys, raw,	182	8%
L	Beef, variety meats and by-products, liver, cooked, braised,	79	3%
L	Beef, variety meats and by-products, liver, cooked, pan-fried,	77	3%
L	Beef, variety meats and by-products, liver, raw,	69	3%
L	Beef, variety meats and by-products, lungs, cooked, braised,	101	4%
M	Beef, variety meats and by-products, lungs, raw,	198	9%
L	Beef, variety meats and by-products, mechanically separated beef, raw,	57	2%
L	Beef, variety meats and by-products, pancreas, cooked, braised,	60	3%
L	Beef, variety meats and by-products, pancreas, raw,	67	3%
L	Beef, variety meats and by-products, spleen, cooked, braised,	57	2%
L	Beef, variety meats and by-products, spleen, raw,	85	4%
L	Beef, variety meats and by-products, thymus, cooked, braised,	116	5%
L	Beef, variety meats and by-products, thymus, raw,	96	4%
L	Beef, variety meats and by-products, tongue, cooked, simmered,	65	3%
L	Beef, variety meats and by-products, tongue, raw,	69	3%
L	Beef, variety meats and by-products, tripe, cooked, simmered,	68	3%
L	Beef, variety meats and by-products, tripe, raw,	97	4%
H	Beet greens, cooked, boiled, drained, with salt,	477	21%

M	Beet greens, cooked, boiled, drained, without salt,	241	10%
M	Beet greens, raw,	226	10%
M	Beets, canned, drained solids,	194	8%
M	Beets, canned, regular pack, solids and liquids,	143	6%
L	Beets, cooked, boiled, drained,	77	3%
M	Beets, cooked, boiled. drained, with salt,	285	12%
M	Beets, harvard, canned, solids and liquids,	162	7%
M	Beets, pickled, canned, solids and liquids,	149	6%
L	Beets, raw,	78	3%
H	Biscuits, mixed grain, refrigerated dough,	670	29%
H	Biscuits, plain or buttermilk, dry mix,	1276	55%
H	Biscuits, plain or buttermilk, dry mix, prepared,	955	42%
H	Biscuits, plain or buttermilk, frozen, baked,	942	41%
H	Biscuits, plain or buttermilk, prepared from recipe,	580	25%
H	Biscuits, plain or buttermilk, refrigerated dough, higher fat,	977	42%
H	Biscuits, plain or buttermilk, refrigerated dough, higher fat, baked,	1002	44%
H	Biscuits, plain or buttermilk, refrigerated dough, lower fat,	828	36%
H	Biscuits, plain or buttermilk, refrigerated dough, lower fat, baked,	962	42%
L	Bison, ground, grass-fed, cooked,	76	3%
L	Bison, ground, grass-fed, raw,	70	3%
L	Blackberries, canned, heavy syrup, solids and liquids,	0	0%
L	Blackberries, frozen, unsweetened,	0	0%
L	Blackberries, raw,	0	0%
L	Blackberry juice, canned,	0	0%
H	Blood sausage,	680	30%
L	Blueberries, canned, heavy syrup, solids and liquids,	0	0%
L	Blueberries, canned, light syrup, drained,	0	0%
L	Blueberries, dried, sweetened,	0	0%
L	Blueberries, frozen, sweetened,	0	0%
L	Blueberries, frozen, unsweetened,	0	0%

L	Blueberries, raw,	0	0%
L	Blueberries, wild, canned, heavy syrup, drained,	0	0%
L	Blueberries, wlld, frozen,	0	0%
H	Bologna, beef,	1013	44%
H	Bologna, beef, low fat,	821	36%
H	Bologna, meat and poultry,	1379	60%
H	Bologna, turkey,	1071	47%
L	Borage, raw,	80	3%
L	Boysenberries, canned, heavy syrup,	0	0%
L	Boysenberries, frozen, unsweetened,	0	0%
L	Bratwurst, chicken, cooked,	72	3%
L	Bratwurst, veal, cooked,	60	3%
H	Bread crumbs, dry, grated, plain,	732	32%
H	Bread crumbs, dry, grated, seasoned,	1336	58%
H	Bread sticks, plain,	713	31%
H	Bread stuffing, bread, dry mix,	1405	61%
H	Bread stuffing, bread, dry mix, prepared,	479	21%
H	Bread stuffing, cornbread, dry mix,	1429	62%
H	Bread stuffing, cornbread, dry mix, prepared,	526	23%
M	Bread, banana, prepared from recipe, made with margarine,	302	13%
H	Bread, boston brown, canned,	631	27%
M	Bread, chapati or roti, plain, commercially prepared,	409	18%
M	Bread, chapati or roti, whole wheat, commercially prepared, frozen,	298	13%
H	Bread, cheese,	750	33%
M	Bread, cinnamon,	388	17%
H	Bread, cornbread, dry mix, enriched (includes corn muffin mix),	817	36%
H	Bread, cornbread, dry mix, prepared with 2% milk, 80% margarine, and eggs,	599	26%
H	Bread, cornbread, dry mix, unenriched (includes corn muffin mix),	1111	48%
H	Bread, cornbread, prepared from recipe, made with low fat (2%) milk,	658	29%
H	Bread, cracked-wheat,	538	23%
M	Bread, egg,	380	17%
M	Bread, egg, toasted,	417	18%

H	Bread, french or vienna (includes sourdough),	602	26%
H	Bread, french or vienna, toasted (includes sourdough),	720	31%
M	Bread, french or vienna, whole wheat,	375	16%
H	Bread, gluten-free, white, made with potato extract, rice starch, and rice flour,	528	23%
M	Bread, gluten-free, white, made with rice flour, corn starch, and\/or tapioca,	447	19%
H	Bread, gluten-free, white, made with tapioca starch and brown rice flour,	515	22%
H	Bread, gluten-free, whole grain, made with tapioca starch and brown rice flour,	510	22%
M	Bread, irish soda, prepared from recipe,	398	17%
H	Bread, italian,	550	24%
L	Bread, kneel down (navajo),	126	5%
M	Bread, multi-grain (includes whole-grain),	381	17%
M	Bread, multi-grain, toasted (includes whole-grain),	414	18%
M	Bread, naan, plain, commercially prepared, refrigerated,	465	20%
M	Bread, naan, whole wheat, commercially prepared, refrigerated,	467	20%
M	Bread, oat bran,	353	15%
M	Bread, oat bran, toasted,	387	17%
M	Bread, oatmeal,	447	19%
H	Bread, oatmeal, toasted,	486	21%
M	Bread, pan dulce, sweet yeast bread,	228	10%
M	Bread, paratha, whole wheat, commercially prepared, frozen,	452	20%
H	Bread, pita, white, enriched,	536	23%
H	Bread, pita, white, unenriched,	536	23%
H	Bread, pita, whole-wheat,	527	23%
M	Bread, potato,	375	16%
M	Bread, pound cake type, pan de torta salvadoran,	390	17%
M	Bread, protein (includes gluten),	404	18%
M	Bread, protein, (includes gluten), toasted,	444	19%
H	Bread, pumpernickel,	596	26%
H	Bread, pumpernickel, toasted,	655	28%
M	Bread, raisin, enriched,	347	15%

M	Bread, raisin, enriched, toasted,	377	16%
M	Bread, raisin, unenriched,	390	17%
M	Bread, reduced-calorie, oat bran,	459	20%
H	Bread, reduced-calorie, oat bran, toasted,	547	24%
M	Bread, reduced-calorie, oatmeal,	388	17%
H	Bread, reduced-calorie, rye,	513	22%
M	Bread, reduced-calorie, wheat,	332	14%
H	Bread, reduced-calorie, white,	479	21%
M	Bread, rice bran,	269	12%
M	Bread, rice bran, toasted,	292	13%
H	Bread, roll, mexican, bollilo,	506	22%
H	Bread, rye,	603	26%
H	Bread, rye, toasted,	664	29%
H	Bread, salvadoran sweet cheese (quesadilla salvadorena),	510	22%
H	Bread, wheat bran,	486	21%
H	Bread, wheat germ, toasted,	621	27%
H	Bread, wheat,	508	22%
H	Bread, wheat, sprouted,	474	21%
H	Bread, wheat, sprouted, toasted,	515	22%
H	Bread, wheat, toasted,	601	26%
H	Bread, white wheat,	478	21%
H	Bread, white, commercially prepared (includes soft bread crumbs),	490	21%
M	Bread, white, commercially prepared, low sodium, no salt,	298	13%
H	Bread, white, commercially prepared, toasted,	537	23%
M	Bread, white, commercially prepared, toasted, low sodium no salt,	376	16%
M	Bread, white, prepared from recipe, made with low fat (2%) milk,	359	16%
M	Bread, white, prepared from recipe, made with nonfat dry milk,	336	15%
M	Bread, whole-wheat, commercially prepared,	455	20%
H	Bread, whole-wheat, commercially prepared, toasted,	565	25%
M	Bread, whole-wheat, prepared from recipe,	346	15%
M	Bread, whole-wheat, prepared from recipe, toasted,	381	17%
L	Breadfruit, raw,	0	0%

M	Breakfast bar, corn flake crust with fruit,	297	13%
M	Breakfast bars, oats, sugar, raisins, coconut (include granola bar),	251	11%
M	Breakfast tart, low fat,	361	16%
M	Broadbeans (fava beans), mature seeds, canned,	453	20%
M	Broadbeans (fava beans), mature seeds, cooked, boiled, with salt,	241	10%
L	Broadbeans (fava beans), mature seeds, cooked, boiled, without salt,	0	0%
L	Broadbeans, immature seeds, raw,	50	2%
L	Broccoli raab, cooked,	56	2%
M	Broccoli, cooked, boiled, drained, with salt,	262	11%
L	Broccoli, cooked, boiled, drained, without salt,	41	2%
M	Broccoli, frozen, chopped, cooked, boiled, drained, with salt,	260	11%
M	Broccoli, frozen, spears, cooked, boiled, drained, with salt,	260	11%
M	Brussels sprouts, cooked, boiled, drained, with salt,	257	11%
M	Brussels sprouts, frozen, cooked, boiled, drained, with salt,	259	11%
L	Buckwheat groats, roasted, cooked,	0	0%
L	Buckwheat,	0	0%
L	Bulgur, cooked,	0	0%
M	Burdock root, cooked, boiled, drained, with salt,	240	10%
L	Burdock root, cooked, boiled, drained, without salt,	0	0%
L	Burdock root, raw,	0	0%
M	Burrito, bean and cheese, frozen,	351	15%
H	Burrito, beef and bean, frozen,	587	26%
H	Burrito, beef and bean, microwaved,	659	29%
L	Butter oil, anhydrous,	0	0%
H	Butter replacement, without fat, powder,	1200	52%
M	Butter, light, stick, with salt,	450	20%
L	Butter, light, stick, without salt,	36	2%
H	Butter, salted,	643	28%
H	Butter, whipped, with salt,	583	25%
L	Butterbur, canned,	0	0%

M	Cabbage, chinese (pak-choi), cooked, boiled, drained, with salt,	270	12%
L	Cabbage, chinese (pak-choi), raw,	65	3%
M	Cabbage, chinese (pe-tsai), cooked, boiled, drained, with salt,	245	11%
M	Cabbage, common, cooked, boiled, drained, with salt,	255	11%
M	Cabbage, japanese style, fresh, pickled,	277	12%
H	Cabbage, kimchi,	498	22%
H	Cabbage, mustard, salted,	717	31%
M	Cabbage, red, cooked, boiled, drained, with salt,	244	11%
M	Cabbage, savoy, cooked, boiled, drained, with salt,	260	11%
H	Cake, angelfood, commercially prepared,	749	33%
H	Cake, angelfood, dry mix,	822	36%
H	Cake, angelfood, dry mix, prepared,	511	22%
M	Cake, boston cream pie, commercially prepared,	254	11%
M	Cake, cherry fudge with chocolate frosting,	164	7%
M	Cake, chocolate, commercially prepared with chocolate frosting, in-store bakery,	348	15%
M	Cake, chocolate, prepared from recipe without frosting,	315	14%
L	Cake, fruitcake, commercially prepared,	101	4%
H	Cake, gingerbread, dry mix,	657	29%
M	Cake, gingerbread, prepared from recipe,	327	14%
M	Cake, pineapple upside-down, prepared from recipe,	319	14%
M	Cake, pound, commercially prepared, butter (includes fresh and frozen),	377	16%
M	Cake, pound, commercially prepared, fat-free,	341	15%
M	Cake, pound, commercially prepared, other than all butter, enriched,	400	17%
M	Cake, pound, commercially prepared, other than all butter, unenriched,	400	17%
H	Cake, pudding-type, carrot, dry mix,	567	25%
H	Cake, pudding-type, chocolate, dry mix,	767	33%
H	Cake, pudding-type, german chocolate, dry mix,	841	37%

H	Cake, pudding-type, marble, dry mix,	519	23%
H	Cake, pudding-type, white, enriched, dry mix,	665	29%
H	Cake, pudding-type, white, unenriched, dry mix,	665	29%
H	Cake, pudding-type, yellow, dry mix,	860	37%
H	Cake, shortcake, biscuit-type, prepared from recipe,	506	22%
M	Cake, snack cakes, creme-filled, chocolate with frosting,	332	14%
H	Cake, snack cakes, creme-filled, chocolate with frosting, low-fat, with added fiber,	483	21%
M	Cake, snack cakes, creme-filled, sponge,	470	20%
M	Cake, snack cakes, not chocolate, with icing or filling, low-fat, with added fiber,	316	14%
H	Cake, sponge, commercially prepared,	623	27%
M	Cake, sponge, prepared from recipe,	228	10%
M	Cake, white, dry mix, special dietary (includes lemon-flavored),	260	11%
M	Cake, white, prepared from recipe with coconut frosting,	284	12%
M	Cake, white, prepared from recipe without frosting,	327	14%
M	Cake, yellow, commercially prepared, with chocolate frosting, in-store bakery,	310	13%
M	Cake, yellow, commercially prepared, with vanilla frosting,	269	12%
H	Cake, yellow, enriched, dry mix,	728	32%
H	Cake, yellow, light, dry mix,	604	26%
M	Cake, yellow, prepared from recipe without frosting,	343	15%
H	Cake, yellow, unenriched, dry mix,	657	29%
L	Canada goose, breast meat, skinless, raw,	50	2%
L	Candies, caramels, chocolate-flavor roll,	44	2%
L	Candies, carob, unsweetened,	107	5%
M	Candies, chocolate covered, caramel with nuts,	156	7%
L	Candies, confectioner's coating, butterscotch,	89	4%
M	Candies, confectioner's coating, peanut butter,	250	11%
L	Candies, confectioner's coating, yogurt,	88	4%

M	Candies, crispy bar with peanut butter filling,	264	11%
L	Candies, fudge, chocolate marshmallow, prepared-from-recipe,	85	4%
L	Candies, fudge, chocolate marshmallow, with nuts, prepared-by-recipe,	79	3%
L	Candies, fudge, chocolate, prepared-from-recipe,	45	2%
L	Candies, fudge, chocolate, with nuts, prepared-from-recipe,	39	2%
L	Candies, fudge, peanut butter, prepared-from-recipe,	118	5%
L	Candies, fudge, vanilla with nuts,	42	2%
L	Candies, fudge, vanilla, prepared-from-recipe,	47	2%
L	Candies, gumdrops, starch jelly pieces,	44	2%
M	Candies, halavah, plain,	195	8%
L	Candies, hard,	38	2%
L	Candies, hard, dietetic or low calorie (sorbitol),	0	0%
L	Candies, marshmallows,	80	3%
L	Candies, milk chocolate coated coffee beans,	70	3%
L	Candies, milk chocolate coated peanuts,	41	2%
L	Candies, milk chocolate,	79	3%
L	Candies, milk chocolate, with almonds,	74	3%
L	Candies, milk chocolate, with rice cereal,	86	4%
M	Candies, peanut bar,	156	7%
M	Candies, peanut brittle, prepared-from-recipe,	445	19%
L	Candles, truffles, prepared-from-recipe,	68	3%
L	Candies, white chocolate,	90	4%
V.H	Capers, canned,	2348	102%
L	Carambola, (starfruit), raw,	0	0%
L	Carbonated chocolate-flavored soda,	0	0%
L	Carbonated, cola, fast-food cola,	0	0%
L	Carbonated, cola, regular,	0	0%
L	Carbonated, cola, without caffeine,	0	0%
L	Carbonated, limeade, high caffeine,	40	2%
L	Carbonated, low calorie, cola or pepper-type, with aspartame, without caffeine,	0	0%
L	Carbonated, reduced sugar, cola, contains caffeine and sweeteners,	0	0%

M	Cardoon, raw,	170	7%
L	Caribou, hind quarter, meat, cooked (alaska native),	45	2%
L	Carissa, (natal-plum), raw,	0	0%
L	Carob-flavor beverage mix, powder,	103	4%
L	Carob-flavor beverage mix, powder, prepared with whole milk,	46	2%
L	Carrot juice, canned,	66	3%
M	Carrot, dehydrated,	275	12%
L	Carrots, baby, raw,	78	3%
L	Carrots, canned, no salt added, drained solids,	42	2%
M	Carrots, canned, regular pack, drained solids,	242	11%
M	Carrots, canned, regular pack, solids and liquids,	240	10%
M	Carrots, cooked, boiled, drained, with salt,	302	13%
L	Carrots, cooked, boiled, drained, without salt,	58	3%
M	Carrots, frozen, cooked, boiled, drained, with salt,	295	13%
L	Carrots, frozen, cooked, boiled, drained, without salt,	59	3%
L	Carrots, frozen, unprepared,	68	3%
L	Carrots, raw,	69	3%
H	Catsup,	907	39%
L	Cattail, narrow leaf shoots (northern plains indians),	109	5%
M	Cauliflower, cooked, boiled, drained, with salt,	242	11%
M	Cauliflower, frozen, cooked, boiled, drained, with salt,	254	11%
M	Cauliflower, green, cooked, with salt,	259	11%
M	Celeriac, cooked, boiled, drained, with salt,	297	13%
L	Celeriac, cooked, boiled, drained, without salt,	61	3%
L	Celeriac, raw,	100	4%
M	Celery, cooked, boiled, drained, with salt,	327	14%
L	Celery, cooked, boiled, drained, without salt,	91	4%
L	Celery, raw,	80	3%
M	Cereals ready-to-eat, wheat and bran, presweetened with nuts and fruits,	245	11%

L	Cereals ready-to-eat, wheat germ, toasted, plain,	0	0%
L	Cereals ready-to-eat, wheat, puffed, fortified,	0	0%
M	Cereals, corn grits, white, regular and quick, enriched, cooked with water, with salt,	223	10%
L	Cereals, corn grits, white, regular and quick, enriched, cooked with water, without salt,	0	0%
L	Cereals, corn grits, white, regular and quick, enriched, dry,	0	0%
L	Cereals, corn grits, yellow, regular and quick, enriched, cooked with water, without salt,	0	0%
L	Cereals, corn grits, yellow, regular and quick, cnrichcd, dry,	0	0%
L	Cereals, corn grits, yellow, regular and quick, unenriched, dry,	0	0%
M	Cereals, corn grits, yellow, regular, quick, enriched, cooked with water, with salt,	223	10%
H	Cereals, oats, instant, fortified, maple and brown sugar, dry,	505	22%
M	Cereals, oats, instant, fortified, plain, dry,	220	10%
L	Cereals, oats, instant, fortified, plain, prepared with water (boiling water added or microwaved),	49	2%
M	Cereals, oats, instant, fortified, with cinnamon and spice, dry,	434	19%
L	Cereals, oats, instant, fortified, with cinnamon and spice, prepared with water,	111	5%
M	Cereals, oats, instant, fortified, with raisins and spice, dry,	462	20%
L	Cereals, oats, instant, fortified, with raisins and spice, prepared with water,	111	5%
L	Cereals, oats, regular and quick and instant, unenriched, cooked with water (includes boiling and microwaving), with salt,	71	3%
L	Cereals, oats, regular and quick, unenriched, cooked with water (includes boiling and microwaving), without salt,	0	0%
M	Cereals, whole wheat hot natural cereal, cooked with water, with salt,	233	10%

L	Cereals, whole wheat hot natural cereal, cooked with water, without salt,	0	0%
L	Cereals, whole wheat hot natural cereal, dry,	0	0%
M	Chard, swiss, cooked, boiled, drained, with salt,	415	18%
M	Chard, swiss, cooked, boiled, drained, without salt,	179	8%
M	Chard, swiss, raw,	213	9%
M	Chayote, fruit, cooked, boiled, drained, with salt,	237	10%
L	Chayote, fruit, cooked, boiled, drained, without salt,	0	0%
L	Chayote, fruit, raw,	0	0%
H	Cheese food, cold pack, american,	966	42%
H	Cheese food, pasteurized process, american, imitation, without added vitamin d,	1297	56%
H	Cheese food, pasteurized process, american, vitamin d fortified,	1284	56%
H	Cheese food, pasteurized process, american, without added vitamin d,	1441	63%
H	Cheese food, pasteurized process, swiss,	1552	67%
H	Cheese product, pasteurized process, american, reduced fat, fortified with vitamin d,	1201	52%
H	Cheese product, pasteurized process, american, vitamin d fortified,	1309	57%
H	Cheese product, pasteurized process, cheddar, reduced fat,	1587	69%
H	Cheese puffs and twists, corn based, baked, low fat,	847	37%
H	Cheese sauce, prepared from recipe,	493	21%
H	Cheese spread, american or cheddar cheese base, reduced fat,	1102	48%
M	Cheese spread, cream cheese base,	436	19%
H	Cheese spread, pasteurized process, american,	1625	71%
H	Cheese substitute, mozzarella,	685	30%
H	Cheese, american cheddar, imitation,	1345	58%
H	Cheese, american, nonfat or fat free,	1316	57%
H	Cheese, blue,	1146	50%
H	Cheese, brick,	560	24%

H	Cheese, brie,	629	27%
H	Cheese, camembert,	842	37%
H	Cheese, caraway,	690	30%
H	Cheese, cheddar,	653	28%
H	Cheese, cheddar, nonfat or fat free,	1000	43%
H	Cheese, cheddar, reduced fat,	628	27%
H	Cheese, cheddar, sharp, sliced,	644	28%
H	Cheese, cheshire,	700	30%
H	Cheese, colby,	604	26%
M	Cheese, cottage, creamed, large or small curd,	364	16%
M	Cheese, cottage, creamed, with fruit,	344	15%
M	Cheese, cottage, lowfat, 1% milkfat,	406	18%
M	Cheese, cottage, lowfat, 1% milkfat, lactose reduced,	220	10%
M	Cheese, cottage, lowfat, 1% milkfat, with vegetables,	403	18%
M	Cheese, cottage, lowfat, 2% milkfat,	308	13%
M	Cheese, cottage, nonfat, uncreamed, dry, large or small curd,	372	16%
M	Cheese, cottage, with vegetables,	403	18%
M	Cheese, cream,	314	14%
H	Cheese, cream, fat free,	702	31%
M	Cheese, cream, low fat,	359	16%
H	Cheese, dry white, queso seco,	1808	79%
H	Cheese, edam,	812	35%
H	Cheese, feta,	917	40%
H	Cheese, fontina,	800	35%
H	Cheese, fresh, queso fresco,	751	33%
H	Cheese, gjetost,	600	26%
M	Cheese, goat, hard type,	423	18%
M	Cheese, goat, semisoft type,	415	18%
M	Cheese, goat, soft type,	459	20%
H	Cheese, gouda,	819	36%
H	Cheese, gruyere,	714	31%
H	Cheese, limburger,	800	35%
H	Cheese, low fat, cheddar or colby,	873	38%
M	Cheese, mexican blend,	338	15%
H	Cheese, mexican, blend, reduced fat,	776	34%
H	Cheese, mexican, queso anejo,	1131	49%

H	Cheese, mexican, queso asadero,	705	31%
H	Cheese, mexican, queso chihuahua,	617	27%
H	Cheese, mexican, queso cotija,	1400	61%
H	Cheese, monterey,	600	26%
H	Cheese, monterey, low fat,	781	34%
H	Cheese, mozzarella, low moisture, part-skim,	666	29%
H	Cheese, mozzarella, low moisture, part-skim, shredded,	682	30%
H	Cheese, mozzarella, nonfat,	743	32%
H	Cheese, mozzarella, part skim milk,	619	27%
H	Cheese, mozzarella, whole milk,	627	27%
H	Cheese, mozzarella, whole milk, low moisture,	710	31%
H	Cheese, muenster,	628	27%
H	Cheese, muenster, low fat,	600	26%
M	Cheese, neufchatel,	334	15%
H	Cheese, parmesan, dry grated, reduced fat,	1529	66%
H	Cheese, parmesan, grated,	1804	78%
H	Cheese, parmesan, hard,	1376	60%
L	Cheese, parmesan, low sodium,	63	3%
H	Cheese, parmesan, shredded,	1696	74%
H	Cheese, pasteurized process, american, fortified with vitamin d,	1671	73%
H	Cheese, pasteurized process, american, low fat,	1789	78%
H	Cheese, pasteurized process, american, without added vitamin d,	1671	73%
H	Cheese, pasteurized process, cheddar or american, fat-free,	1528	66%
H	Cheese, pasteurized process, pimento,	915	40%
H	Cheese, pasteurized process, swiss,	1370	60%
H	Cheese, pasteurized process, swiss, low fat,	1430	62%
H	Cheese, port de salut,	534	23%
H	Cheese, provolone,	876	38%
H	Cheese, provolone, reduced fat,	615	27%
L	Cheese, ricotta, part skim milk,	99	4%
L	Cheese, ricotta, whole milk,	84	4%
H	Cheese, romano,	1433	62%
H	Cheese, roquefort,	1809	79%
M	Cheese, swiss,	187	8%

M	Cheese, swiss, low fat,	199	9%
H	Cheese, swiss, nonfat or fat free,	1000	43%
H	Cheese, tilsit,	753	33%
H	Cheese, white, queso blanco,	704	31%
M	Cheesecake commercially prepared,	438	19%
M	Cheesecake prepared from mix, no-bake type,	380	17%
L	Cherries, sour, canned, water pack, drained,	0	0%
L	Cherries, sour, red, frozen, unsweetened,	0	0%
L	Cherries, sour, red, raw,	0	0%
L	Cherries, sweet, canned, extra heavy syrup pack, solids and liquids,	0	0%
L	Cherries, sweet, canned, juice pack, solids and liquids,	0	0%
L	Cherries, sweet, canned, light syrup pack, solids and liquids,	0	0%
L	Cherries, sweet, canned, pitted, heavy syrup pack, solids and liquids,	0	0%
L	Cherries, sweet, canned, pitted, heavy syrup, drained,	0	0%
L	Cherries, sweet, canned, water pack, solids and liquids,	0	0%
L	Cherries, sweet, frozen, sweetened,	0	0%
L	Cherries, sweet, raw,	0	0%
L	Chewing gum,	0	0%
M	Chicken breast tenders, breaded, cooked, microwaved,	446	19%
H	Chicken breast tenders, breaded, uncooked,	536	23%
H	Chicken breast, deli, rotisserie seasoned, sliced, prepackaged,	1032	45%
H	Chicken breast, fat-free, mesquite flavor, sliced,	1040	45%
H	Chicken breast, oven-roasted, fat-free, sliced,	1087	47%
H	Chicken patty, frozen, cooked,	532	23%
H	Chicken patty, frozen, uncooked,	518	23%
M	Chicken pot pie, frozen entree, prepared,	393	17%
H	Chicken spread,	722	31%
H	Chicken tenders, breaded, frozen, prepared,	527	23%
L	Chicken, broiler or fryers, breast, skinless, boneless, meat only, cooked, braised,	47	2%

L	Chicken, broiler or fryers, breast, skinless, boneless, meat only, cooked, grilled,	52	2%
L	Chicken, broiler or fryers, breast, skinless, boneless, meat only, raw,	45	2%
M	Chicken, broiler or fryers, breast, skinless, boneless, meat only, with added solution, cooked, braised,	172	7%
M	Chicken, broiler or fryers, breast, skinless, boneless, meat only, with added solution, cooked, grilled,	215	9%
H	Chicken, broiler, rotisserie, bbq, back meat and skin,	509	22%
H	Chicken, broiler, rotisserie, bbq, back meat only,	563	24%
M	Chicken, broiler, rotisserie, bbq, breast meat and skin,	329	14%
M	Chicken, broiler, rotisserie, bbq, breast meat only,	328	14%
M	Chicken, broiler, rotisserie, bbq, drumstick meat and skin,	392	17%
M	Chicken, broiler, rotisserie, bbq, drumstick, meat only,	403	18%
M	Chicken, broiler, rotisserie, bbq, skin,	335	15%
M	Chicken, broiler, rotisserie, bbq, thigh meat and skin,	335	15%
M	Chicken, broiler, rotisserie, bbq, thigh, meat only,	335	15%
H	Chicken, broiler, rotisserie, bbq, wing meat and skin,	579	25%
H	Chicken, broiler, rotisserie, bbq, wing, meat only,	725	32%
M	Chicken, broilers or fryers, back, meat and skin, cooked, fried, batter,	317	14%
L	Chicken, broilers or fryers, back, meat and skin, cooked, fried, flour,	90	4%
L	Chicken, broilers or fryers, back, meat and skin, cooked, roasted,	87	4%
H	Chicken, broilers or fryers, back, meat and skin, cooked, rotisserie, original seasoning,	584	25%

L	Chicken, broilers or fryers, back, meat and skin, cooked, stewed,	64	3%
L	Chicken, broilers or fryers, back, meat and skin, raw,	64	3%
L	Chicken, broilers or fryers, back, meat only, cooked, fried,	99	4%
L	Chicken, broilers or fryers, back, meat only, cooked, roasted,	96	4%
H	Chicken, broilers or fryers, back, meat only, cooked, rotisserie, original seasoning,	661	29%
L	Chicken, broilers or fryers, back, meat only, cooked, stewed,	67	3%
L	Chicken, broilers or fryers, back, meat only, raw,	82	4%
M	Chicken, broilers or fryers, breast, meat and skin, cooked, fried, batter,	275	12%
L	Chicken, broilers or fryers, breast, meat and skin, cooked, fried, flour,	76	3%
L	Chicken, broilers or fryers, breast, meat and skin, cooked, roasted,	71	3%
M	Chicken, broilers or fryers, breast, meat and skin, cooked, rotisserie, original seasoning,	347	15%
L	Chicken, broilers or fryers, breast, meat and skin, cooked, stewed,	62	3%
L	Chicken, broilers or fryers, breast, meat and skin, raw,	63	3%
L	Chicken, broilers or fryers, breast, meat only, cooked, fried,	79	3%
L	Chicken, broilers or fryers, breast, meat only, cooked, roasted,	74	3%
M	Chicken, broilers or fryers, breast, meat only, cooked, rotisserie, original seasoning,	313	14%
L	Chicken, broilers or fryers, breast, meat only, cooked, stewed,	63	3%
M	Chicken, broilers or fryers, breast, skinless, boneless, meat only, with added solution, raw,	173	8%
L	Chicken, broilers or fryers, dark meat, drumstick, meat and skin, cooked, braised,	111	5%

L	Chicken, broilers or fryers, dark meat, drumstick, meat only, cooked, braised,	117	5%
M	Chicken, broilers or fryers, dark meat, drumstick, meat only, cooked, roasted,	128	6%
L	Chicken, broilers or fryers, dark meat, drumstick, meat only, raw,	114	5%
M	Chicken, broilers or fryers, dark meat, meat and skin, cooked, fried, batter,	295	13%
L	Chicken, broilers or fryers, dark meat, meat and skin, cooked, fried, flour,	89	4%
L	Chicken, broilers or fryers, dark meat, meat and skin, cooked, roasted,	87	4%
L	Chicken, broilers or fryers, dark meat, meat and skin, cooked, stewed,	70	3%
L	Chicken, broilers or fryers, dark meat, meat and skin, raw,	73	3%
L	Chicken, broilers or fryers, dark meat, meat only, cooked, fried,	97	4%
L	Chicken, broilers or fryers, dark meat, meat only, cooked, roasted,	93	4%
L	Chicken, broilers or fryers, dark meat, meat only, cooked, stewed,	74	3%
L	Chicken, broilers or fryers, dark meat, meat only, raw,	85	4%
L	Chicken, broilers or fryers, dark meat, thigh, meat and skin, cooked, braised,	76	3%
L	Chicken, broilers or fryers, dark meat, thigh, meat only, cooked, braised,	77	3%
L	Chicken, broilers or fryers, dark meat, thigh, meat only, raw,	95	4%
M	Chicken, broilers or fryers, drumstick, meat and skin, cooked, fried, batter,	269	12%
L	Chicken, broilers or fryers, drumstick, meat and skin, cooked, fried, flour,	89	4%
L	Chicken, broilers or fryers, drumstick, meat and skin, cooked, roasted,	123	5%
M	Chicken, broilers or fryers, drumstick, meat and skin, cooked, rotisserie, original seasoning,	411	18%

L	Chicken, broilers or fryers, drumstick, meat and skin, cooked, stewed,	76	3%
L	Chicken, broilers or fryers, drumstick, meat and skin, raw,	106	5%
L	Chicken, broilers or fryers, drumstick, meat only, cooked, fried,	96	4%
M	Chicken, broilers or fryers, drumstick, meat only, cooked, rotisserie, original seasoning,	417	18%
L	Chicken, broilers or fryers, drumstick, meat only, cooked, stewed,	80	3%
L	Chicken, broilers or fryers, giblets, cooked, fried,	113	5%
L	Chicken, broilers or fryers, giblets, cooked, simmered,	67	3%
L	Chicken, broilers or fryers, giblets, raw,	77	3%
M	Chicken, broilers or fryers, leg, meat and skin, cooked, fried, batter,	279	12%
L	Chicken, broilers or fryers, leg, meat and skin, cooked, fried, flour,	88	4%
L	Chicken, broilers or fryers, leg, meat and skin, cooked, roasted,	98	4%
L	Chicken, broilers or fryers, leg, meat and skin, cooked, stewed,	73	3%
L	Chicken, broilers or fryers, leg, meat and skin, raw,	84	4%
L	Chicken, broilers or fryers, leg, meat only, cooked, fried,	96	4%
L	Chicken, broilers or fryers, leg, meat only, cooked, roasted,	99	4%
L	Chicken, broilers or fryers, leg, meat only, cooked, stewed,	78	3%
L	Chicken, broilers or fryers, leg, meat only, raw,	96	4%
M	Chicken, broilers or fryers, light meat, meat and skin, cooked, fried, batter,	287	12%
L	Chicken, broilers or fryers, light meat, meat and skin, cooked, fried, flour,	77	3%
L	Chicken, broilers or fryers, light meat, meat and skin, cooked, roasted,	75	3%

L	Chicken, broilers or fryers, light meat, meat and skin, cooked, stewed,	63	3%
L	Chicken, broilers or fryers, light meat, meat and skin, raw,	65	3%
L	Chicken, broilers or fryers, light meat, meat only, cooked, fried,	81	4%
L	Chicken, broilers or fryers, light meat, meat only, cooked, roasted,	77	3%
L	Chicken, broilers or fryers, light meat, meat only, cooked, stewed,	65	3%
L	Chicken, broilers or fryers, light meat, meat only, raw,	68	3%
M	Chicken, broilers or fryers, meat and skin and giblets and neck, cooked, fried, batter,	284	12%
L	Chicken, broilers or fryers, meat and skin and giblets and neck, cooked, fried, flour,	86	4%
L	Chicken, broilers or fryers, meat and skin and giblets and neck, raw,	70	3%
L	Chicken, broilers or fryers, meat and skin and giblets and neck, roasted,	79	3%
L	Chicken, broilers or fryers, meat and skin and giblets and neck, stewed,	66	3%
M	Chicken, broilers or fryers, meat and skin, cooked, fried, batter,	292	13%
L	Chicken, broilers or fryers, meat and skin, cooked, fried, flour,	84	4%
L	Chicken, broilers or fryers, meat and skin, cooked, roasted,	82	4%
L	Chicken, broilers or fryers, meat and skin, cooked, stewed,	67	3%
L	Chicken, broilers or fryers, meat and skin, raw,	70	3%
L	Chicken, broilers or fryers, meat only, cooked, fried,	91	4%
L	Chicken, broilers or fryers, meat only, raw,	77	3%
L	Chicken, broilers or fryers, meat only, roasted,	86	4%
L	Chicken, broilers or fryers, meat only, stewed,	70	3%
L	Chicken, broilers or fryers, neck, meat and skin, cooked simmered,	52	2%

M	Chicken, broilers or fryers, neck, meat and skin, cooked, fried, batter,	276	12%
L	Chicken, broilers or fryers, neck, meat and skin, cooked, fried, flour,	82	4%
L	Chicken, broilers or fryers, neck, meat and skin, raw,	64	3%
L	Chicken, broilers or fryers, neck, meat only, cooked, fried,	99	4%
L	Chicken, broilers or fryers, neck, meat only, cooked, simmered,	64	3%
L	Chicken, broilers or fryers, neck, meat only, raw,	81	4%
H	Chicken, broilers or fryers, skin only, cooked, fried, batter,	581	25%
L	Chicken, broilers or fryers, skin only, cooked, fried, flour,	53	2%
L	Chicken, broilers or fryers, skin only, cooked, roasted,	65	3%
M	Chicken, broilers or fryers, skin only, cooked, rotisserie, original seasoning,	381	17%
L	Chicken, broilers or fryers, skin only, cooked, stewed,	56	2%
L	Chicken, broilers or fryers, skin only, raw,	63	3%
M	Chicken, broilers or fryers, thigh, meat and skin, cooked, fried, batter,	288	13%
L	Chicken, broilers or fryers, thigh, meat and skin, cooked, fried, flour,	88	4%
L	Chicken, broilers or fryers, thigh, meat and skin, cooked, roasted,	102	4%
M	Chicken, broilers or fryers, thigh, meat and skin, cooked, rotisserie, original seasoning,	345	15%
L	Chicken, broilers or fryers, thigh, meat and skin, cooked, stewed,	71	3%
L	Chicken, broilers or fryers, thigh, meat and skin, raw,	81	4%
L	Chicken, broilers or fryers, thigh, meat only, cooked, fried,	95	4%
L	Chicken, broilers or fryers, thigh, meat only, cooked, roasted,	106	5%

M	Chicken, broilers or fryers, thigh, meat only, cooked, rotisserie, original seasoning,	337	15%
L	Chicken, broilers or fryers, thigh, meat only, cooked, stewed,	75	3%
M	Chicken, broilers or fryers, wing, meat and skin, cooked, fried, batter,	320	14%
L	Chicken, broilers or fryers, wing, meat and skin, cooked, fried, flour,	77	3%
L	Chicken, broilers or fryers, wing, meat and skin, cooked, roasted,	98	4%
H	Chicken, broilers or fryers, wing, meat and skin, cooked, rotisserie, original seasoning,	610	27%
L	Chicken, broilers or fryers, wing, meat and skin, cooked, stewed,	67	3%
L	Chicken, broilers or fryers, wing, meat and skin, raw,	84	4%
L	Chicken, broilers or fryers, wing, meat only, cooked, fried,	91	4%
L	Chicken, broilers or fryers, wing, meat only, cooked, roasted,	92	4%
H	Chicken, broilers or fryers, wing, meat only, cooked, rotisserie, original seasoning,	725	32%
L	Chicken, broilers or fryers, wing, meat only, cooked, stewed,	73	3%
L	Chicken, broilers or fryers, wing, meat only, raw,	81	4%
H	Chicken, canned, meat only, with broth,	503	22%
H	Chicken, canned, no broth,	482	21%
L	Chicken, capons, giblets, cooked, simmered,	55	2%
L	Chicken, capons, giblets, raw,	77	3%
L	Chicken, capons, meat and skin and giblets and neck, cooked, roasted,	50	2%
L	Chicken, capons, meat and skin and giblets and neck, raw,	47	2%
L	Chicken, capons, meat and skin, cooked, roasted,	49	2%
L	Chicken, capons, meat and skin, raw,	45	2%
L	Chicken, cornish game hens, meat and skin, cooked, roasted,	64	3%

L	Chicken, cornish game hens, meat and skin, raw,	61	3%
L	Chicken, cornish game hens, meat only, cooked, roasted,	63	3%
L	Chicken, cornish game hens, meat only, raw,	68	3%
M	Chicken, dark meat, drumstick, meat and skin, with added solution, cooked, braised,	165	7%
M	Chicken, dark meat, drumstick, meat and skin, with added solution, cooked, roasted,	186	8%
M	Chicken, dark meat, drumstick, meat and skin, with added solution, raw,	150	7%
M	Chicken, dark meat, drumstick, meat only, with added solution, cooked, braised,	169	7%
M	Chicken, dark meat, drumstick, meat only, with added solution, cooked, roasted,	190	8%
M	Chicken, dark meat, drumstick, meat only, with added solution, raw,	152	7%
M	Chicken, dark meat, thigh, meat and skin, with added solution, cooked, braised,	185	8%
M	Chicken, dark meat, thigh, meat and skin, with added solution, cooked, roasted,	174	8%
M	Chicken, dark meat, thigh, meat and skin, with added solution, raw,	151	7%
M	Chicken, dark meat, thigh, meat only, with added solution, cooked, braised,	197	9%
M	Chicken, dark meat, thigh, meat only, with added solution, cooked, roasted,	177	8%
M	Chicken, dark meat, thigh, meat only, with added solution, raw,	156	7%
L	Chicken, feet, boiled,	67	3%
L	Chicken, gizzard, all classes, cooked, simmered,	56	2%
L	Chicken, gizzard, all classes, raw,	69	3%
L	Chicken, ground, crumbles, cooked, pan-browned,	75	3%
L	Chicken, ground, raw,	60	3%
L	Chicken, heart, all classes, cooked, simmered,	48	2%
L	Chicken, heart, all classes, raw,	74	3%
L	Chicken, liver, all classes, cooked, pan-fried,	92	4%

L	Chicken, liver, all classes, cooked, simmered,	76	3%
L	Chicken, liver, all classes, raw,	71	3%
H	Chicken, meatless,	709	31%
M	Chicken, meatless, breaded, fried,	400	17%
H	Chicken, nuggets, dark and white meat, precooked, frozen, not reheated,	560	24%
H	Chicken, nuggets, white meat, precooked, frozen, not reheated,	538	23%
L	Chicken, roasting, dark meat, meat only, cooked, roasted,	95	4%
L	Chicken, roasting, dark meat, meat only, raw,	95	4%
L	Chicken, roasting, giblets, cooked, simmered,	60	3%
L	Chicken, roasting, giblets, raw,	77	3%
L	Chicken, roasting, light meat, meat only, cooked, roasted,	51	2%
L	Chicken, roasting, light meat, meat only, raw,	51	2%
L	Chicken, roasting, meat and skin and giblets and neck, cooked, roasted,	71	3%
L	Chicken, roasting, meat and skin and giblets and neck, raw,	69	3%
L	Chicken, roasting, meat and skin, cooked, roasted,	73	3%
L	Chicken, roasting, meat only, cooked, roasted,	75	3%
L	Chicken, roasting, meat only, raw,	75	3%
L	Chicken, skin (drumsticks and thighs), cooked, braised,	75	3%
L	Chicken, skin (drumsticks and thighs), cooked, roasted,	85	4%
L	Chicken, skin (drumsticks and thighs), raw,	51	2%
M	Chicken, skin (drumsticks and thighs), with added solution, cooked, braised,	139	6%
M	Chicken, skin (drumsticks and thighs), with added solution, cooked, roasted,	162	7%
M	Chicken, skin (drumsticks and thighs), with added solution, raw,	139	6%
L	Chicken, stewing, dark meat, meat only, cooked, stewed,	95	4%
L	Chicken, stewing, dark meat, meat only, raw,	101	4%
L	Chicken, stewing, giblets, cooked, simmered,	56	2%

L	Chicken, stewing, giblets, raw,	77	3%
L	Chicken, stewing, light meat, meat only, cooked, stewed,	58	3%
L	Chicken, stewing, light meat, meat only, raw,	53	2%
L	Chicken, stewing, meat and skin, and giblets and neck, cooked, stewed,	67	3%
L	Chicken, stewing, meat and skin, and giblets and neck, raw,	71	3%
L	Chicken, stewing, meat and skin, cooked, stewed,	73	3%
L	Chicken, stewing, meat and skin, raw,	71	3%
L	Chicken, stewing, meat only, cooked, stewed,	78	3%
L	Chicken, stewing, meat only, raw,	79	3%
H	Chicken, thighs, frozen, breaded, reheated,	813	35%
H	Chicken, wing, frozen, glazed, barbecue flavored,	615	27%
H	Chicken, wing, frozen, glazed, barbecue flavored, heated (conventional oven),	559	24%
H	Chicken, wing, frozen, glazed, barbecue flavored, heated (microwave),	837	36%
L	Chickpea flour (besan),	64	3%
M	Chickpeas (garbanzo beans, bengal gram), mature seeds, canned, drained solids,	246	11%
M	Chickpeas (garbanzo beans, bengal gram), mature seeds, canned, drained, rinsed in tap water,	212	9%
M	Chickpeas (garbanzo beans, bengal gram), mature seeds, canned, solids and liquids,	278	12%
M	Chickpeas (garbanzo beans, bengal gram), mature seeds, canned, solids and liquids, low sodium,	132	6%
M	Chickpeas (garbanzo beans, bengal gram), mature seeds, cooked, boiled, with salt,	243	11%
L	Chicory greens, raw,	45	2%
L	Chicory roots, raw,	50	2%
L	Chicory, witloof, raw,	0	0%
M	Chili con carne with beans, canned entree,	449	20%
M	Chili with beans, canned,	423	18%
M	Chili with beans, microwavable bowls,	385	17%
M	Chili, no beans, canned entree,	411	18%

L	Chives, freeze-dried,	70	3%
L	Chives, raw,	0	0%
L	Chocolate almond milk, unsweetened, shelf-stable, fortified with vitamin d2 and e,	75	3%
L	Chocolate drink, milk and soy based, ready to drink, fortified,	63	3%
L	Chocolate malt powder, prepared with 1% milk, fortified,	60	3%
L	Chocolate malt, powder, prepared with fat free milk,	77	3%
H	Chocolate powder, no sugar added,	636	28%
L	Chocolate syrup,	72	3%
L	Chocolate syrup, prepared with whole milk,	47	2%
M	Chocolate-flavor beverage mix for milk, powder, with added nutrients,	136	6%
L	Chocolate-flavor beverage mix for milk, powder, with added nutrients, prepared with whole milk,	50	2%
L	Chocolate-flavor beverage mix, powder, prepared with whole milk,	58	3%
L	Chocolate-flavored drink, whey and milk based,	91	4%
L	Chocolate-flavored hazelnut spread,	41	2%
L	Chokecherries, raw, pitted (northern plains indians),	0	0%
L	Chrysanthemum leaves, raw,	118	5%
M	Chrysanthemum, garland, cooked, boiled, drained, with salt,	289	13%
L	Chrysanthemum, garland, cooked, boiled, drained, without salt,	53	2%
L	Chrysanthemum, garland, raw,	118	5%
M	Cinnamon buns, frosted (includes honey buns),	305	13%
L	Citrus fruit juice drink, frozen concentrate,	0	0%
L	Citrus fruit juice drink, frozen concentrate, prepared with water,	0	0%
M	Clam and tomato juice, canned,	362	16%
L	Clementines, raw,	0	0%
L	Cocktail mix, non-alcoholic, concentrated, frozen,	0	0%

H	Cocoa mix, low calorie, powder, with added calcium, phosphorus, aspartame, without added sodium or vitamin a,	653	28%
H	Cocoa mix, nestle, rich chocolate hot cocoa mix,	850	37%
H	Cocoa mix, no sugar added, powder,	876	38%
H	Cocoa mix, powder,	504	22%
L	Cocoa mix, powder, prepared with water,	73	3%
L	Cocoa mix, with aspartame, powder, prepared with water,	72	3%
L	Cocoa, dry powder, unsweetened, hershey's european style cocoa,	0	0%
H	Coffee and cocoa, instant, decaffeinated, with whitener and low calorie sweetener,	500	22%
L	Coffee substitute, cereal grain powder,	83	4%
L	Coffee substitute, cereal grain powder, prepared with whole milk,	49	2%
L	Coffee substitute, cereal grain prepared with water,	0	0%
L	Coffee, brewed, breakfast blend,	0	0%
L	Coffee, brewed, prepared with tap water,	0	0%
L	Coffee, brewed, prepared with tap water, decaffeinated,	0	0%
L	Coffee, instant, decaffeinated, prepared with water,	0	0%
M	Coffee, instant, mocha, sweetened,	317	14%
L	Coffee, instant, regular, half the caffeine,	37	2%
L	Coffee, instant, regular, powder,	37	2%
L	Coffee, instant, regular, prepared with water,	0	0%
M	Coffee, instant, vanilla, sweetened, decaffeinated, with non dairy creamer,	333	14%
M	Coffee, instant, with chicory,	277	12%
L	Coffee, instant, with whitener, reduced calorie,	0	0%
M	Coffeecake, cheese,	339	15%
M	Coffeecake, cinnamon with crumb topping, commercially prepared, enriched,	351	15%
M	Coffeecake, cinnamon with crumb topping, commercially prepared, unenriched,	351	15%

H	Coffeecake, cinnamon with crumb topping, dry mix,	596	26%
M	Coffeecake, cinnamon with crumb topping, dry mix, prepared,	421	18%
M	Coffeecake, creme-filled with chocolate frosting,	323	14%
M	Coffeecake, fruit,	385	17%
M	Collards, cooked, boiled, drained, with salt,	252	11%
M	Collards, frozen, chopped, cooked, boiled, drained, with salt,	286	12%
L	Collards, frozen, chopped, cooked, boiled, drained, without salt,	50	2%
L	Collards, frozen, chopped, unprepared,	48	2%
M	Cookie, butter or sugar, with chocolate icing or filling,	348	15%
M	Cookie, chocolate, with icing or coating,	380	17%
M	Cookie, vanilla with caramel, coconut, and chocolate coating,	182	8%
M	Cookie, with peanut butter filling, chocolate-coated,	371	16%
M	Cookies, animal crackers (includes arrowroot, tea biscuits),	407	18%
M	Cookies, animal, with frosting or icing,	257	11%
M	Cookies, brownies, commercially prepared,	286	12%
M	Cookies, brownies, commercially prepared, reduced fat, with added fiber,	290	13%
M	Cookies, brownies, dry mix, regular,	303	13%
L	Cookies, brownies, dry mix, sugar free,	83	4%
M	Cookies, brownies, prepared from recipe,	343	15%
M	Cookies, butter, commercially prepared, enriched,	282	12%
M	Cookies, butter, commercially prepared, unenriched,	351	15%
M	Cookies, chocolate chip sandwich, with creme filling,	279	12%
M	Cookies, chocolate chip, commercially prepared, regular, higher fat, enriched,	311	14%
M	Cookies, chocolate chip, commercially prepared, regular, higher fat, unenriched,	315	14%

M	Cookies, chocolate chip, commercially prepared, regular, lower fat,	418	18%
M	Cookies, chocolate chip, commercially prepared, soft-type,	276	12%
M	Cookies, chocolate chip, commercially prepared, special dietary,	244	11%
M	Cookies, chocolate chip, dry mix,	290	13%
M	Cookies, chocolate chip, prepared from recipe, made with butter,	341	15%
M	Cookies, chocolate chip, prepared from recipe, made with margarine,	361	16%
M	Cookies, chocolate chip, refrigerated dough,	321	14%
M	Cookies, chocolate chip, refrigerated dough, baked,	232	10%
M	Cookies, chocolate cream covered biscuit sticks,	213	9%
M	Cookies, chocolate sandwich, with creme filling, reduced fat,	471	20%
M	Cookies, chocolate sandwich, with creme filling, regular,	388	17%
M	Cookies, chocolate sandwich, with creme filling, regular, chocolate-coated,	326	14%
M	Cookies, chocolate sandwich, with creme filling, special dietary,	342	15%
M	Cookies, chocolate sandwich, with extra creme filling,	351	15%
H	Cookies, chocolate wafers,	580	25%
M	Cookies, chocolate, made with rice cereal,	210	9%
M	Cookies, coconut macaroon,	241	10%
M	Cookies, fig bars,	350	15%
M	Cookies, fudge, cake-type (includes trolley cakes),	192	8%
H	Cookies, gingersnaps,	501	22%
M	Cookies, gluten-free, chocolate sandwich, with creme filling,	275	12%
L	Cookies, gluten-free, chocolate wafer,	122	5%
L	Cookies, gluten-free, lemon wafer,	111	5%
M	Cookies, gluten-free, vanilla sandwich, with creme filling,	201	9%

M	Cookies, ladyfingers, with lemon juice and rind,	147	6%
M	Cookies, ladyfingers, without lemon juice and rind,	147	6%
M	Cookies, marie biscuit,	370	16%
M	Cookies, marshmallow, chocolate-coated (includes marshmallow pies),	188	8%
M	Cookies, marshmallow, with rice cereal and chocolate chips,	341	15%
M	Cookies, molasses,	459	20%
M	Cookies, oatmeal sandwich, with creme filling,	444	19%
M	Cookies, oatmeal, commercially prepared, regular,	383	17%
M	Cookies, oatmeal, commercially prepared, soft-type,	349	15%
M	Cookies, oatmeal, commercially prepared, special dietary,	273	12%
H	Cookies, oatmeal, dry mix,	473	21%
H	Cookies, oatmeal, prepared from recipe, with raisins,	538	23%
H	Cookies, oatmeal, prepared from recipe, without raisins,	598	26%
H	Cookies, oatmeal, reduced fat,	562	24%
M	Cookies, oatmeal, refrigerated dough,	294	13%
M	Cookies, oatmeal, refrigerated dough, baked,	327	14%
M	Cookies, peanut butter sandwich, regular,	368	16%
M	Cookies, peanut butter sandwich, special dietary,	412	18%
M	Cookies, peanut butter, commercially prepared, regular,	463	20%
M	Cookies, peanut butter, commercially prepared, soft-type,	336	15%
M	Cookies, peanut butter, commercially prepared, sugar free,	448	19%
H	Cookies, peanut butter, prepared from recipe,	518	23%
M	Cookies, peanut butter, refrigerated dough,	397	17%
M	Cookies, peanut butter, refrigerated dough, baked,	436	19%
M	Cookies, raisin, soft-type,	418	18%

M	Cookies, shortbread, commercially prepared, pecan,	281	12%
M	Cookies, shortbread, commercially prepared, plain,	353	15%
H	Cookies, shortbread, reduced fat,	571	25%
M	Cookies, sugar wafer, chocolate-covered,	138	6%
L	Cookies, sugar wafer, with creme filling, sugar free,	71	3%
L	Cookies, sugar wafers with creme filling, regular,	103	4%
M	Cookies, sugar, commercially prepared, regular (includes vanilla),	385	17%
H	Cookies, sugar, prepared from recipe, made with margarine,	491	21%
M	Cookies, sugar, refrigerated dough,	328	14%
M	Cookies, sugar, refrigerated dough, baked,	362	16%
M	Cookies, vanilla sandwich with creme filling,	349	15%
M	Cookies, vanilla sandwich with creme filling, reduced fat,	354	15%
M	Cookies, vanilla wafers, higher fat,	325	14%
M	Cookies, vanilla wafers, lower fat,	388	17%
L	Coriander (cilantro) leaves, raw,	46	2%
H	Corn dogs, frozen, prepared,	668	29%
L	Corn flour, masa, enriched, white,	0	0%
L	Corn flour, masa, unenriched, white,	0	0%
L	Corn flour, whole-grain, blue (harina de maiz morado),	0	0%
L	Corn flour, whole-grain, white,	0	0%
L	Corn flour, whole-grain, yellow,	0	0%
L	Corn flour, yellow, degermed, unenriched,	0	0%
L	Corn flour, yellow, masa, enriched,	0	0%
M	Corn pudding, home prepared,	282	12%
M	Corn with red and green peppers, canned, solids and liquids,	347	15%
L	Corn, dried, yellow (northern plains indians),	0	0%
L	Corn, sweet, white, canned, cream style, no salt added,	0	0%
M	Corn, sweet, white, canned, cream style, regular pack,	261	11%

L	Corn, sweet, white, canned, vacuum pack, no salt added,	0	0%
M	Corn, sweet, white, canned, vacuum pack, regular pack,	272	12%
M	Corn, sweet, white, canned, whole kernel, drained solids,	185	8%
M	Corn, sweet, white, canned, whole kernel, regular pack, solids and liquids,	213	9%
M	Corn, sweet, white, cooked, boiled, drained, with salt,	253	11%
L	Corn, sweet, white, cooked, boiled, drained, without salt,	0	0%
M	Corn, sweet, white, frozen, kernels cut off cob, boiled, drained, with salt,	245	11%
L	Corn, sweet, white, frozen, kernels cut off cob, boiled, drained, without salt,	0	0%
L	Corn, sweet, white, frozen, kernels cut off cob, unprepared,	0	0%
M	Corn, sweet, white, frozen, kernels on cob, cooked, boiled, drained, with salt,	240	10%
L	Corn, sweet, white, frozen, kernels on cob, cooked, boiled, drained, without salt,	0	0%
L	Corn, sweet, white, frozen, kernels on cob, unprepared,	0	0%
M	Corn, sweet, yellow, canned, brine pack, regular pack, solids and liquids,	195	8%
L	Corn, sweet, yellow, canned, cream style, no salt added,	0	0%
M	Corn, sweet, yellow, canned, cream style, regular pack,	261	11%
M	Corn, sweet, yellow, canned, drained solids, rinsed with tap water,	163	7%
L	Corn, sweet, yellow, canned, vacuum pack, no salt added,	0	0%
M	Corn, sweet, yellow, canned, vacuum pack, regular pack,	272	12%
M	Corn, sweet, yellow, canned, whole kernel, drained solids,	205	9%
M	Corn, sweet, yellow, cooked, boiled, drained, with salt,	253	11%

L	Corn, sweet, yellow, cooked, boiled, drained, without salt,	0	0%
L	Corn, sweet, yellow, frozen, kernels cut off cob, boiled, drained, without salt,	0	0%
L	Corn, sweet, yellow, frozen, kernels cut off cob, unprepared,	0	0%
M	Corn, sweet, yellow, frozen, kernels on cob, cooked, boiled, drained, with salt,	240	10%
L	Corn, sweet, yellow, frozen, kernels on cob, cooked, boiled, drained, without salt,	0	0%
L	Corn, sweet, yellow, frozen, kernels on cob, unprepared,	0	0%
M	Corn, sweet, yellow, frozen, kernels, cut off cob, boiled, drained, with salt,	245	11%
L	Corn, yellow, whole kernel, frozen, microwaved,	0	0%
H	Corned beef loaf, jellied,	953	41%
H	Cornmeal, white, self-rising, bolted, plain, enriched,	1247	54%
H	Cornmeal, white, self-rising, bolted, with wheat flour added, enriched,	1319	57%
H	Cornmeal, white, self-rising, degermed, enriched,	1348	59%
H	Cornmeal, yellow, self-rising, bolted, plain, enriched,	1247	54%
H	Cornmeal, yellow, self-rising, bolted, with wheat flour added, enriched,	1319	57%
H	Cornmeal, yellow, self-rising, degermed, enriched,	1348	59%
L	Cornsalad, raw,	0	0%
L	Couscous, cooked,	0	0%
M	Cowpeas (blackeyes), immature seeds, cooked, boiled, drained, with salt,	240	10%
L	Cowpeas (blackeyes), immature seeds, cooked, boiled, drained, without salt,	0	0%
M	Cowpeas (blackeyes), immature seeds, frozen, cooked, boiled, drained, with salt,	241	10%
L	Cowpeas (blackeyes), immature seeds, frozen, cooked, boiled, drained, without salt,	0	0%
L	Cowpeas (blackeyes), immature seeds, raw,	0	0%

M	Cowpeas, catjang, mature seeds, cooked, boiled, with salt,	255	11%
L	Cowpeas, catjang, mature seeds, raw,	58	3%
M	Cowpeas, common (blackeyes, crowder, southern), mature seeds, canned, plain,	293	13%
M	Cowpeas, common (blackeyes, crowder, southern), mature seeds, cooked, boiled, with salt,	240	10%
L	Cowpeas, common (blackeyes, crowder, southern), mature seeds, cooked, boiled, without salt,	0	0%
M	Cowpeas, leafy tips, cooked, boiled, drained, with salt,	242	11%
M	Cowpeas, young pods with seeds, cooked, boiled, drained, with salt,	239	10%
L	Cowpeas, young pods with seeds, cooked, boiled, drained, without salt,	0	0%
L	Cowpeas, young pods with seeds, raw,	0	0%
L	Crabapples, raw,	0	0%
M	Crackers, cheese, low sodium,	458	20%
H	Crackers, cheese, reduced fat,	1167	51%
H	Crackers, cheese, regular,	973	42%
H	Crackers, cheese, sandwich-type with cheese filling,	878	38%
H	Crackers, cheese, sandwich-type with peanut butter filling,	829	36%
H	Crackers, cheese, whole grain,	802	35%
M	Crackers, crispbread, rye,	410	18%
H	Crackers, flavored, fish-shaped,	970	42%
M	Crackers, gluten-free, multi-seeded and multigrain,	438	19%
H	Crackers, gluten-free, multigrain and vegetable, made with corn starch and white rice flour,	890	39%
M	Crackers, matzo, egg and onion,	285	12%
L	Crackers, matzo, plain,	0	0%
L	Crackers, matzo, whole-wheat,	0	0%
H	Crackers, melba toast, plain,	598	26%
H	Crackers, melba toast, rye (includes pumpernickel),	899	39%

H	Crackers, melba toast, wheat,	837	36%
H	Crackers, milk,	687	30%
H	Crackers, multigrain,	883	38%
M	Crackers, rusk toast,	253	11%
H	Crackers, rye, sandwich-type with cheese filling,	1044	45%
H	Crackers, rye, wafers, plain,	557	24%
H	Crackers, rye, wafers, seasoned,	887	39%
H	Crackers, saltines (includes oyster, soda, soup),	941	41%
H	Crackers, saltines, fat-free, low-sodium,	849	37%
M	Crackers, saltines, low salt (includes oyster, soda, soup),	198	9%
H	Crackers, saltines, unsalted tops (includes oyster, soda, soup),	766	33%
H	Crackers, saltines, whole wheat (includes multi-grain),	1214	53%
H	Crackers, sandwich-type, peanut butter filled, reduced fat,	639	28%
H	Crackers, snack, goya crackers,	665	29%
H	Crackers, standard snack-type, regular,	726	32%
M	Crackers, standard snack-type, regular, low salt,	216	9%
H	Crackers, standard snack-type, sandwich, with cheese filling,	978	43%
H	Crackers, standard snack-type, sandwich, with peanut butter filling,	801	35%
H	Crackers, standard snack-type, with whole wheat,	748	33%
M	Crackers, toast thins, low sodium,	177	8%
H	Crackers, water biscuits,	571	25%
M	Crackers, wheat, low salt,	190	8%
H	Crackers, wheat, reduced fat,	776	34%
H	Crackers, wheat, regular,	699	30%
H	Crackers, wheat, sandwich, with cheese filling,	839	36%
H	Crackers, wheat, sandwich, with peanut butter filling,	807	35%
H	Crackers, whole grain, sandwich-type, with peanut butter filling,	635	28%

H	Crackers, whole-wheat,	704	31%
M	Crackers, whole-wheat, low salt,	186	8%
H	Crackers, whole-wheat, reduced fat,	745	32%
L	Cranberries, dried, sweetened,	0	0%
L	Cranberries, raw,	0	0%
L	Cranberry juice cocktail,	0	0%
L	Cranberry juice cocktail, bottled,	0	0%
L	Cranberry juice cocktail, bottled, low calorie, with calcium, saccharin and corn sweetener,	0	0%
L	Cranberry juice cocktail, frozen concentrate,	0	0%
L	Cranberry juice cocktail, frozen concentrate, prepared with water,	0	0%
L	Cranberry juice, unsweetened,	0	0%
L	Cranberry sauce, canned, sweetened,	0	0%
L	Cranberry-apple juice drink, bottled,	0	0%
L	Cranberry-apple juice drink, low calorie, with vitamin c added,	0	0%
L	Cranberry-apricot juice drink, bottled,	0	0%
L	Cranberry-grape juice drink, bottled,	0	0%
H	Cream puff shell, prepared from recipe,	483	21%
M	Cream puff, eclair, custard or cream filled, iced,	265	12%
L	Cream substitute, flavored, liquid,	67	3%
L	Cream substitute, flavored, powdered,	123	5%
L	Cream substitute, liquid, light,	60	3%
L	Cream substitute, liquid, with hydrogenated vegetable oil and soy protein,	67	3%
L	Cream substitute, liquid, with lauric acid oil and sodium caseinate,	79	3%
L	Cream substitute, powdered,	124	5%
M	Cream substitute, powdered, light,	229	10%
L	Cream, fluid, half and half,	61	3%
L	Cream, fluid, light (coffee cream or table cream),	72	3%
L	Cream, half and half, fat free,	100	4%
L	Cream, sour, reduced fat, cultured,	89	4%
H	Creamy dressing, made with sour cream and\/or buttermilk and oil, reduced calorie,	833	36%

H	Creamy dressing, made with sour cream and\/or buttermilk and oil, reduced calorie, cholesterol-free,	932	41%
H	Creamy dressing, made with sour cream and\/or buttermilk and oil, reduced calorie, fat-free,	897	39%
M	Cress, garden, cooked, boiled, drained, with salt,	244	11%
M	Croissants, apple,	274	12%
M	Croissants, butter,	467	20%
M	Croissants, cheese,	361	16%
H	Croutons, plain,	698	30%
H	Croutons, seasoned,	1089	47%
H	Crustaceans, crab, alaska king, cooked, moist heat,	1072	47%
H	Crustaceans, crab, alaska king, imitation, made from surimi,	529	23%
H	Crustaceans, crab, alaska king, raw,	836	36%
H	Crustaceans, crab, blue, canned,	563	24%
M	Crustaceans, crab, blue, cooked, moist heat,	395	17%
M	Crustaceans, crab, blue, crab cakes, home recipe,	330	14%
M	Crustaceans, crab, blue, raw,	293	13%
M	Crustaceans, crab, dungeness, cooked, moist heat,	378	16%
M	Crustaceans, crab, dungeness, raw,	295	13%
H	Crustaceans, crab, queen, cooked, moist heat,	691	30%
H	Crustaceans, crab, queen, raw,	539	23%
L	Crustaceans, crayfish, mixed species, farmed, cooked, moist heat,	97	4%
L	Crustaceans, crayfish, mixed species, farmed, raw,	62	3%
L	Crustaceans, crayfish, mixed species, wild, cooked, moist heat,	94	4%
L	Crustaceans, crayfish, mixed species, wild, raw,	58	3%
H	Crustaceans, lobster, northern, cooked, moist heat,	486	21%
M	Crustaceans, lobster, northern, raw,	423	18%

L	Crustaceans, shrimp, cooked (not previously frozen),	111	5%
H	Crustaceans, shrimp, mixed species, canned,	870	38%
M	Crustaceans, shrimp, mixed species, cooked, breaded and fried,	344	15%
H	Crustaceans, shrimp, mixed species, cooked, moist heat (may have been previously frozen),	947	41%
H	Crustaceans, shrimp, mixed species, imitation, made from surimi,	705	31%
H	Crustaceans, shrimp, mixed species, raw (may have been previously frozen),	566	25%
L	Crustaceans, shrimp, raw (not previously frozen),	119	5%
M	Crustaceans, spiny lobster, mixed species, cooked, moist heat,	227	10%
M	Crustaceans, spiny lobster, mixed species, raw,	177	8%
L	Cucumber, peeled, raw,	0	0%
L	Cucumber, with peel, raw,	0	0%
L	Currants, european black, raw,	0	0%
L	Currants, red and white, raw,	0	0%
L	Dairy drink mix, chocolate, reduced calorie, with aspartame, powder, prepared with water and ice,	61	3%
H	Dairy drink mix, chocolate, reduced calorie, with low-calorie sweeteners, powder,	659	29%
M	Dandelion greens, cooked, boiled, drained, with salt,	280	12%
L	Dandelion greens, cooked, boiled, drained, without salt,	44	2%
L	Dandelion greens, raw,	76	3%
M	Danish pastry, cheese,	417	18%
M	Danish pastry, cinnamon, enriched,	414	18%
M	Danish pastry, cinnamon, unenriched,	371	16%
M	Danish pastry, fruit, enriched (includes apple, cinnamon, raisin, lemon, raspberry, strawberry),	445	19%
M	Danish pastry, fruit, unenriched (includes apple, cinnamon, raisin, strawberry),	354	15%

M	Danish pastry, lemon, unenriched,	354	15%
M	Danish pastry, nut (includes almond, raisin nut, cinnamon nut),	298	13%
M	Danish pastry, raspberry, unenriched,	354	15%
L	Dates, deglet noor,	0	0%
L	Dates, medjool,	0	0%
L	Dessert topping, powdered, 1.5 ounce prepared with 1V2 cup milk,	66	3%
L	Dessert topping, pressurized,	62	3%
L	Desserts, egg custard, baked, prepared-from-recipe,	61	3%
L	Desserts, flan, caramel custard, prepared-from-recipe,	53	2%
L	Desserts, mousse, chocolate, prepared-from-recipe,	38	2%
L	Dill weed, fresh,	61	3%
M	Doughnuts, cake-type, chocolate, sugared or glazed,	215	9%
H	Doughnuts, cake-type, plain (includes unsugared, old-fashioned),	477	21%
M	Doughnuts, cake-type, plain, chocolate-coated or frosted,	326	14%
M	Doughnuts, cake-type, plain, sugared or glazed,	402	17%
M	Doughnuts, french crullers, glazed,	345	15%
M	Doughnuts, yeast-leavened, glazed, enriched (includes honey buns),	316	14%
M	Doughnuts, yeast-leavened, glazed, unenriched (includes honey buns),	342	15%
M	Doughnuts, yeast-leavened, with creme filling,	309	13%
M	Doughnuts, yeast-leavened, with jelly filling,	455	20%
L	Dove, cooked (includes squab),	57	2%
H	Dressing, honey mustard, fat-free,	1004	44%
M	Drumstick leaves, cooked, boiled, drained, with salt,	245	11%
M	Drumstick pods, cooked, boiled, drained, with salt,	279	12%
L	Drumstick pods, cooked, boiled, drained, without salt,	43	2%

L	Drumstick pods, raw,	42	2%
M	Duck, domesticated, liver, raw,	140	6%
L	Duck, domesticated, meat and skin, cooked, roasted,	59	3%
L	Duck, domesticated, meat and skin, raw,	63	3%
L	Duck, domesticated, meat only, cooked, roasted,	65	3%
L	Duck, domesticated, meat only, raw,	74	3%
L	Duck, wild, breast, meat only, raw,	57	2%
L	Duck, wild, meat and skin, raw,	56	2%
L	Duck, young duckling, domesticated, white pekin, breast, meat and skin, boneless, cooked, roasted,	84	4%
L	Duck, young duckling, domesticated, white pekin, breast, meat only, boneless, cooked without skin, broiled,	105	5%
L	Duck, young duckling, domesticated, white pekin, leg, meat and skin, bone in, cooked, roasted,	110	5%
L	Duck, young duckling, domesticated, white pekin, leg, meat only, bone in, cooked without skin, braised,	108	5%
M	Dulce de leche,	129	6%
H	Dumpling, potato- or cheese-filled, frozen,	474	21%
L	Durian, raw or frozen,	0	0%
M	Egg custards, dry mix,	281	12%
L	Egg custards, dry mix, prepared with 2% milk,	87	4%
L	Egg custards, dry mix, prepared with whole milk,	84	4%
H	Egg rolls, chicken, refrigerated, heated,	478	21%
H	Egg rolls, vegetable, frozen, prepared,	490	21%
M	Egg substitute, liquid or frozen, fat free,	199	9%
H	Egg substitute, powder,	800	35%
M	Egg, duck, whole, fresh, raw,	146	6%
M	Egg, goose, whole, fresh, raw,	138	6%
M	Egg, quail, whole, fresh, raw,	141	6%
M	Egg, turkey, whole, fresh, raw,	151	7%
H	Egg, white, dried,	1280	56%
H	Egg, white, dried, flakes, stabilized, glucose reduced,	1156	50%

H	Egg, white, dried, powder, stabilized, glucose reduced,	1238	54%
H	Egg, white, dried, stabilized, glucose reduced,	1299	56%
M	Egg, white, raw, fresh,	166	7%
M	Egg, white, raw, frozen, pasteurized,	169	7%
M	Egg, whole, cooked, fried,	207	9%
L	Egg, whole, cooked, hard-boiled,	124	5%
M	Egg, whole, cooked, omelet,	155	7%
M	Egg, whole, cooked, poached,	297	13%
M	Egg, whole, cooked, scrambled,	145	6%
H	Egg, whole, dried,	476	21%
H	Egg, whole, dried, stabilized, glucose reduced,	548	24%
M	Egg, whole, raw, fresh,	142	6%
M	Egg, whole, raw, frozen, pasteurized,	128	6%
V.H	Egg, whole, raw, frozen, salted, pasteurized,	3663	159%
M	Egg, yolk, dried,	149	6%
L	Egg, yolk, raw, fresh,	48	2%
L	Egg, yolk, raw, frozen, pasteurized,	67	3%
V.H	Egg, yolk, raw, frozen, salted, pasteurized,	3487	152%
L	Egg, yolk, raw, frozen, sugared, pasteurized,	70	3%
L	Eggnog-flavor mix, powder, prepared with whole milk,	55	2%
L	Eggnog,	54	2%
M	Eggplant, cooked, boiled, drained, with salt,	239	10%
L	Eggplant, cooked, boiled, drained, without salt,	0	0%
H	Eggplant, pickled,	1674	73%
L	Eggplant, raw,	0	0%
M	Eggs, scrambled, frozen mixture,	162	7%
L	Emu, fan fillet, cooked, broiled,	53	2%
L	Emu, fan fillet, raw,	120	5%
M	Emu, flat fillet, raw,	150	7%
L	Emu, full rump, cooked, broiled,	110	5%
L	Emu, full rump, raw,	90	4%
L	Emu, ground, cooked, pan-broiled,	65	3%
L	Emu, ground, raw,	56	2%
L	Emu, inside drum, raw,	102	4%
L	Emu, inside drums, cooked, broiled,	118	5%

L	Emu, outside drum, raw,	100	4%
M	Emu, oyster, raw,	150	7%
L	Emu, top loin, cooked, broiled,	58	3%
L	Energy drink with carbonated water and high fructose corn syrup,	48	2%
L	Energy drink, monster, fortified with vitamins c, b2, b3, b6, b12,	77	3%
L	Energy drink, sugar free,	42	2%
M	English muffins, mixed-grain (includes granola),	298	13%
M	English muffins, mixed-grain, toasted (includes granola),	324	14%
M	English muffins, plain, enriched, with ca prop (includes sourdough),	425	18%
M	English muffins, plain, enriched, without calcium propionate(includes sourdough),	464	20%
H	English muffins, plain, toasted, enriched, with calcium propionate (includes sourdough),	477	21%
M	English muffins, plain, unenriched, with calcium propionate (includes sourdough),	464	20%
M	English muffins, plain, unenriched, without calcium propionate (includes sourdough),	464	20%
M	English muffins, raisin-cinnamon (includes apple-cinnamon),	299	13%
M	English muffins, raisin-cinnamon, toasted (includes apple-cinnamon),	342	15%
M	English muffins, wheat,	353	15%
M	English muffins, wheat, toasted,	384	17%
M	English muffins, whole grain white,	386	17%
M	English muffins, whole-wheat,	364	16%
M	English muffins, whole-wheat, toasted,	396	17%
L	Epazote, raw,	43	2%
M	Falafel, home-prepared,	294	13%
H	Fast food, biscuit,	979	43%
H	Fast food, pizza chain, 1/4 pizza, cheese topping, regular crust,	598	26%
H	Fast food, pizza chain, 1/4 pizza, cheese topping, stuffed crust,	615	27%
H	Fast food, pizza chain, 1/4 pizza, cheese topping, thick crust,	597	26%

H	Fast food, pizza chain, 1/4 pizza, cheese topping, thin crust,	742	32%
H	Fast food, pizza chain, 1/4 pizza, meat and vegetable topping, regular crust,	589	26%
H	Fast food, pizza chain, 1/4 pizza, pepperoni topping, regular crust,	685	30%
H	Fast food, pizza chain, 1/4 pizza, pepperoni topping, thin crust,	875	38%
H	Fast food, pizza chain, 1/4 pizza, sausage topping, regular crust,	633	28%
H	Fast food, pizza chain, 1/4 pizza, sausage topping, thick crust,	637	28%
H	Fast food, pizza chain, 1/4 pizza, sausage topping, thin crust,	782	34%
H	Fast food, pizza chain, 1/4pizza, pepperoni topping, thick crust,	684	30%
H	Fast foods, bagel, with breakfast steak, egg, cheese, and condiments,	642	28%
H	Fast foods, bagel, with egg, sausage patty, cheese, and condiments,	550	24%
H	Fast foods, biscuit with egg and steak,	600	26%
H	Fast foods, biscuit, with crispy chicken fillet,	868	38%
H	Fast foods, biscuit, with egg and sausage,	672	29%
H	Fast foods, biscuit, with egg,	655	28%
H	Fast foods, biscuit, with sausage,	814	35%
H	Fast foods, breadstick, soft, prepared with garlic and parmesan cheese,	539	23%
H	Fast foods, breakfast burrito, with egg, cheese, and sausage,	744	32%
H	Fast foods, burrito, with beans and beef,	570	25%
H	Fast foods, burrito, with beans and cheese,	563	24%
M	Fast foods, burrito, with beans,	454	20%
M	Fast foods, burrito, with beans, cheese, and beef,	451	20%
H	Fast foods, cheeseburger, double, regular patty and bun, with condiments,	617	27%
M	Fast foods, cheeseburger; double, large patty, with condiments and vegetables,	445	19%
H	Fast foods, cheeseburger; double, large patty; with condiments,	480	21%

M	Fast foods, cheeseburger; double, large patty; with condiments, vegetables and mayonnaise,	405	18%
H	Fast foods, cheeseburger; double, regular patty, with condiments and vegetables,	633	28%
H	Fast foods, cheeseburger; double, regular patty; double decker bun with condiments and special sauce,	485	21%
H	Fast foods, cheeseburger; double, regular patty; plain,	621	27%
H	Fast foods, cheeseburger; double, regular patty; with condiments,	617	27%
M	Fast foods, cheeseburger; double, regular, patty and bun; with condiments and vegetables,	404	18%
H	Fast foods, cheeseburger; single, large patty; plain,	481	21%
M	Fast foods, cheeseburger; single, large patty; with condiments and vegetables,	385	17%
H	Fast foods, cheeseburger; single, large patty; with condiments,	591	26%
H	Fast foods, cheeseburger; single, large patty; with condiments, vegetables and mayonnaise,	473	21%
H	Fast foods, cheeseburger; single, regular patty, with condiments and vegetables,	546	24%
H	Fast foods, cheeseburger; single, regular patty, with condiments,	628	27%
H	Fast foods, cheeseburger; single, regular patty; plain,	515	22%
H	Fast foods, cheeseburger; triple, regular patty; plain,	637	28%
H	Fast foods, chicken fillet sandwich, plain with pickles,	753	33%
H	Fast foods, chicken tenders,	769	33%
H	Fast foods, chicken, breaded and fried, boneless pieces, plain,	594	26%
M	Fast foods, coleslaw,	203	9%
H	Fast foods, crispy chicken filet sandwich, with lettuce and mayonnaise,	617	27%

H	Fast foods, crispy chicken in tortilla, with lettuce, cheese, and ranch sauce,	607	26%
M	Fast foods, croissant, with egg and cheese,	434	19%
H	Fast foods, croissant, wlth egg, cheese, and sausage,	577	25%
M	Fast foods, egg, scrambled,	187	8%
H	Fast foods, english muffin, with cheese and sausage,	668	29%
H	Fast foods, english muffin, with egg, cheese, and sausage,	548	24%
M	Fast foods, fish sandwich, with tartar sauce and cheese,	434	19%
H	Fast foods, fish sandwich, with tartar sauce,	602	26%
M	Fast foods, french toast sticks,	400	17%
M	Fast foods, french toast with butter,	380	17%
H	Fast foods, fried chicken, breast, meat and skin and breading,	657	29%
H	Fast foods, fried chicken, breast, meat only, skin and breading removed,	512	22%
H	Fast foods, fried chicken, drumstick, meat and skin with breading,	591	26%
H	Fast foods, fried chicken, drumstick, meat only, skin and breading removed,	492	21%
H	Fast foods, fried chicken, thigh, meat and skin and breading,	747	32%
H	Fast foods, fried chicken, thigh, meat only, skin and breading removed,	577	25%
H	Fast foods, fried chicken, wing, meat and skin and breading,	867	38%
H	Fast foods, fried chicken, wing, meat only, skin and breading removed,	761	33%
H	Fast foods, griddle cake sandwich, egg, cheese, and sausage,	652	28%
H	Fast foods, griddle cake sandwich, sausage,	737	32%
M	Fast foods, grilled chicken filet sandwich, with lettuce, tomato and spread,	427	19%
H	Fast foods, grilled chicken in tortilla, with lettuce, cheese, and ranch sauce,	577	25%
H	Fast foods, hotdog, plain,	684	30%
M	Fast foods, hotdog, with chili,	421	18%

H	Fast foods, hotdog, with corn flour coating (corndog),	556	24%
H	Fast foods, hush puppies,	813	35%
H	Fast foods, miniature cinnamon rolls,	554	24%
M	Fast foods, nachos, with cheese,	313	14%
M	Fast foods, nachos, with cheese, beans, ground beef, and tomatoes,	348	15%
H	Fast foods, onion rings, breaded and fried,	776	34%
M	Fast foods, potato, french fried in vegetable oil,	210	9%
M	Fast foods, potato, mashed,	306	13%
H	Fast foods, potatoes, hash browns, round pieces or patty,	566	25%
H	Fast foods, quesadilla, with chicken,	745	32%
H	Fast foods, roast beef sandwich, plain,	653	28%
H	Fast foods, shrimp, breaded and fried,	897	39%
H	Fast foods, submarine sandwich, cold cut on white bread with lettuce and tomato,	575	25%
M	Fast foods, submarine sandwich, meatball marinara on white bread,	437	19%
M	Fast foods, submarine sandwich, oven roasted chicken on white bread with lettuce and tomato,	268	12%
M	Fast foods, submarine sandwich, roast beef on white bread with lettuce and tomato,	329	14%
M	Fast foods, submarine sandwich, steak and cheese on white bread with cheese, lettuce and tomato,	444	19%
M	Fast foods, submarine sandwich, sweet onion chicken teriyaki on white bread with lettuce, tomato and sweet onion sauce,	305	13%
M	Fast foods, submarine sandwich, tuna on white bread with lettuce and tomato,	329	14%
M	Fast foods, submarine sandwich, turkey breast on white bread with lettuce and tomato,	317	14%
L	Fast foods, sundae, caramel,	126	5%
L	Fast foods, sundae, hot fudge,	115	5%
L	Fast foods, sundae, strawberry,	60	3%
M	Fast foods, taco salad,	385	17%

M	Fast foods, taco with beef, cheese and lettuce, hard shell,	397	17%
H	Fast foods, taco with beef, cheese and lettuce, soft,	560	24%
H	Fast foods, taco with chicken, lettuce and cheese, soft,	613	27%
L	Fast foods, vanilla, light, soft-serve ice cream, with cone,	81	4%
L	Fat free ice cream, no sugar added, flavors other than chocolate,	110	5%
L	Fat, beef tallow,	0	0%
L	Fat, chicken,	0	0%
L	Fat, duck,	0	0%
L	Fat, goose,	0	0%
L	Fat, mutton tallow,	0	0%
L	Fat, turkey,	0	0%
L	Feijoa, raw,	0	0%
L	Fennel, bulb, raw,	52	2%
L	Figs, canned, extra heavy syrup pack, solids and liquids,	0	0%
L	Figs, canned, heavy syrup pack, solids and liquids,	0	0%
L	Figs, canned, light syrup pack, solids and liquids,	0	0%
L	Figs, canned, water pack, solids and liquids,	0	0%
L	Figs, dried, stewed,	0	0%
L	Figs, raw,	0	0%
M	Fish broth,	318	14%
L	Fish oil, cod liver,	0	0%
L	Fish oil, herring,	0	0%
L	Fish oil, menhaden,	0	0%
L	Fish oil, menhaden, fully hydrogenated,	0	0%
L	Fish oil, salmon,	0	0%
L	Fish oil, sardine,	0	0%
V.H	Fish, anchovy, european, canned in oil, drained solids,	3668	159%
L	Fish, anchovy, european, raw,	104	5%
L	Fish, bass, fresh water, mixed species, raw,	70	3%
L	Fish, bass, freshwater, mixed species, cooked, dry heat,	90	4%

L	Fish, bass, striped, cooked, dry heat,	88	4%
L	Fish, bass, striped, raw,	69	3%
L	Fish, bluefish, cooked, dry heat,	77	3%
L	Fish, bluefish, raw,	60	3%
L	Fish, burbot, cooked, dry heat,	124	5%
L	Fish, burbot, raw,	97	4%
L	Fish, butterfish, cooked, dry heat,	114	5%
L	Fish, butterfish, raw,	89	4%
L	Fish, carp, cooked, dry heat,	63	3%
L	Fish, carp, raw,	49	2%
M	Fish, catfish, channel, cooked, breaded and fried,	280	12%
L	Fish, catfish, channel, farmed, cooked, dry heat,	119	5%
L	Fish, catfish, channel, farmed, raw,	98	4%
L	Fish, catfish, channel, wild, cooked, dry heat,	50	2%
L	Fish, catfish, channel, wild, raw,	43	2%
H	Fish, caviar, black and red, granular,	1500	65%
L	Fish, cisco, raw,	55	2%
H	Fish, cisco, smoked,	481	21%
M	Fish, cod, atlantic, canned, solids and liquid,	218	9%
L	Fish, cod, atlantic, cooked, dry heat,	78	3%
V.H	Fish, cod, atlantic, dried and salted,	7027	306%
L	Fish, cod, atlantic, raw,	54	2%
M	Fish, cod, pacific, cooked (not previously frozen),	134	6%
M	Fish, cod, pacific, cooked, dry heat (may have been previously frozen),	372	16%
M	Fish, cod, pacific, raw (may have been previously frozen),	303	13%
L	Fish, cod, pacific, raw (not previously frozen),	109	5%
M	Fish, croaker, atlantic, cooked, breaded and fried,	348	15%
L	Fish, croaker, atlantic, raw,	56	2%
L	Fish, cusk, cooked, dry heat,	40	2%
L	Fish, drum, freshwater, cooked, dry heat,	96	4%
L	Fish, drum, freshwater, raw,	75	3%
L	Fish, eel, mixed species, cooked, dry heat,	65	3%
L	Fish, eel, mixed species, raw,	51	2%

M	Fish, fish sticks, frozen, prepared,	402	17%
M	Fish, flatfish (flounder and sole species), cooked, dry heat,	363	16%
M	Fish, flatfish (flounder and sole species), raw,	296	13%
H	Fish, gefiltefish, commercial, sweet recipe,	524	23%
L	Fish, grouper, mixed species, cooked, dry heat,	53	2%
L	Fish, grouper, mixed species, raw,	53	2%
M	Fish, haddock, cooked, dry heat,	261	11%
M	Fish, haddock, raw,	213	9%
H	Fish, haddock, smoked,	763	33%
L	Fish, halibut, atlantic and pacific, cooked, dry heat,	82	4%
L	Fish, halibut, atlantic and pacific, raw,	68	3%
L	Fish, halibut, greenland, cooked, dry heat,	103	4%
L	Fish, halibut, greenland, raw,	80	3%
L	Fish, herring, atlantic, cooked, dry heat,	115	5%
H	Fish, herring, atlantic, kippered,	918	40%
H	Fish, herring, atlantic, pickled,	870	38%
L	Fish, herring, atlantic, raw,	90	4%
L	Fish, herring, pacific, cooked, dry heat,	95	4%
L	Fish, herring, pacific, raw,	74	3%
M	Fish, ling, cooked, dry heat,	173	8%
M	Fish, ling, raw,	135	6%
L	Fish, lingcod, cooked, dry heat,	76	3%
L	Fish, lingcod, raw,	59	3%
L	Fish, mackerel, atlantic, cooked, dry heat,	83	4%
L	Fish, mackerel, atlantic, raw,	90	4%
M	Fish, mackerel, jack, canned, drained solids,	379	16%
M	Fish, mackerel, king, cooked, dry heat,	203	9%
M	Fish, mackerel, king, raw,	158	7%
L	Fish, mackerel, pacific and jack, mixed species, cooked, dry heat,	110	5%
L	Fish, mackerel, pacific and jack, mixed species, raw,	86	4%
V.H	Fish, mackerel, salted,	4450	193%
L	Fish, mackerel, spanish, cooked, dry heat,	66	3%
L	Fish, mackerel, spanish, raw,	59	3%
L	Fish, mahimahi, cooked, dry heat,	113	5%

L	Fish, mahimahi, raw,	88	4%
L	Fish, milkfish, cooked, dry heat,	92	4%
L	Fish, milkfish, raw,	72	3%
L	Fish, mullet, striped, cooked, dry heat,	71	3%
L	Fish, mullet, striped, raw,	65	3%
M	Fish, ocean perch, atlantic, cooked, dry heat,	347	15%
M	Fish, ocean perch, atlantic, raw,	287	12%
L	Fish, perch, mixed species, cooked, dry heat,	79	3%
L	Fish, perch, mixed species, raw,	62	3%
L	Fish, pike, northern, cooked, dry heat,	49	2%
L	Fish, pike, northern, raw,	39	2%
L	Fish, pike, walleye, cooked, dry heat,	65	3%
L	Fish, pike, walleye, raw,	51	2%
M	Fish, pollock, alaska, cooked (not previously frozen),	166	7%
M	Fish, pollock, alaska, cooked, dry heat (may have been previously frozen),	419	18%
M	Fish, pollock, alaska, raw (may have been previously frozen),	333	14%
M	Fish, pollock, alaska, raw (not previously frozen),	159	7%
L	Fish, pollock, atlantic, cooked, dry heat,	110	5%
L	Fish, pollock, atlantic, raw,	86	4%
L	Fish, pompano, florida, cooked, dry heat,	76	3%
L	Fish, pompano, florida, raw,	65	3%
L	Fish, pout, ocean, cooked, dry heat,	78	3%
L	Fish, pout, ocean, raw,	61	3%
L	Fish, rockfish, pacific, mixed species, cooked, dry heat,	89	4%
L	Fish, rockfish, pacific, mixed species, raw,	74	3%
L	Fish, roe, mixed species, cooked, dry heat,	117	5%
L	Fish, roe, mixed species, raw,	91	4%
L	Fish, roughy, orange, cooked, dry heat,	69	3%
L	Fish, roughy, orange, raw,	72	3%
L	Fish, sablefish, cooked, dry heat,	72	3%
L	Fish, sablefish, raw,	56	2%
H	Fish, sablefish, smoked,	737	32%
L	Fish, salmon, atlantic, farmed, cooked, dry heat,	61	3%

L	Fish, salmon, atlantic, farmed, raw,	59	3%
L	Fish, salmon, atlantic, wild, cooked, dry heat,	56	2%
L	Fish, salmon, atlantic, wild, raw,	44	2%
L	Fish, salmon, chinook, cooked, dry heat,	60	3%
L	Fish, salmon, chinook, raw,	47	2%
H	Fish, salmon, chinook, smoked,	672	29%
H	Fish, salmon, chinook, smoked, (lox), regular,	2000	87%
M	Fish, salmon, chum, canned, drained solids with bone,	391	17%
L	Fish, salmon, chum, canned, without salt, drained solids with bone,	75	3%
L	Fish, salmon, chum, cooked, dry heat,	64	3%
L	Fish, salmon, chum, raw,	50	2%
L	Fish, salmon, coho, farmed, cooked, dry heat,	52	2%
L	Fish, salmon, coho, farmed, raw,	47	2%
L	Fish, salmon, coho, wild, cooked, dry heat,	58	3%
L	Fish, salmon, coho, wild, cooked, moist heat,	53	2%
L	Fish, salmon, coho, wild, raw,	46	2%
M	Fish, salmon, pink, canned, drained solids,	381	17%
M	Fish, salmon, pink, canned, drained solids, without skin and bones,	378	16%
M	Fish, salmon, pink, canned, total can contents,	403	18%
L	Fish, salmon, pink, canned, without salt, solids with bone and liquid,	75	3%
L	Fish, salmon, pink, cooked, dry heat,	90	4%
L	Fish, salmon, pink, raw,	75	3%
M	Fish, salmon, sockeye, canned, drained solids,	408	18%
L	Fish, salmon, sockeye, canned, without salt, drained solids with bone,	75	3%
L	Fish, salmon, sockeye, cooked, dry heat,	92	4%
L	Fish, salmon, sockeye, raw,	78	3%
M	Fish, sardine, atlantic, canned in oil, drained solids with bone,	307	13%
M	Fish, sardine, pacific, canned in tomato sauce, drained solids with bone,	414	18%
L	Fish, scup, cooked, dry heat,	54	2%
L	Fish, scup, raw,	42	2%

L	Fish, sea bass, mixed species, cooked, dry heat,	87	4%
L	Fish, sea bass, mixed species, raw,	68	3%
L	Fish, seatrout, mixed species, cooked, dry heat,	74	3%
L	Fish, seatrout, mixed species, raw,	58	3%
L	Fish, shad, american, cooked, dry heat,	65	3%
L	Fish, shad, american, raw,	51	2%
L	Fish, shark, mixed species, cooked, batter-dipped and fried,	122	5%
L	Fish, shark, mixed species, raw,	79	3%
L	Fish, sheepshead, cooked, dry heat,	73	3%
L	Fish, sheepshead, raw,	71	3%
L	Fish, smelt, rainbow, cooked, dry heat,	77	3%
L	Fish, smelt, rainbow, raw,	60	3%
L	Fish, snapper, mixed species, cooked, dry heat,	57	2%
L	Fish, snapper, mixed species, raw,	64	3%
L	Fish, spot, cooked, dry heat,	37	2%
L	Fish, sturgeon, mixed species, cooked, dry heat,	69	3%
L	Fish, sturgeon, mixed species, raw,	54	2%
H	Fish, sturgeon, mixed species, smoked,	739	32%
L	Fish, sucker, white, cooked, dry heat,	51	2%
L	Fish, sucker, white, raw,	40	2%
L	Fish, sunfish, pumpkin seed, cooked, dry heat,	103	4%
L	Fish, sunfish, pumpkin seed, raw,	80	3%
M	Fish, surimi,	143	6%
L	Fish, swordfish, cooked, dry heat,	97	4%
L	Fish, swordfish, raw,	81	4%
L	Fish, tilapia, cooked, dry heat,	56	2%
L	Fish, tilapia, raw,	52	2%
L	Fish, tilefish, cooked, dry heat,	59	3%
L	Fish, tilefish, raw,	53	2%
L	Fish, trout, brook, raw, new york state,	45	2%
L	Fish, trout, mixed species, cooked, dry heat,	67	3%
L	Fish, trout, mixed species, raw,	52	2%

L	Fish, trout, rainbow, farmed, cooked, dry heat,	61	3%
L	Fish, trout, rainbow, farmed, raw,	51	2%
L	Fish, trout, rainbow, wild, cooked, dry heat,	56	2%
M	Fish, tuna salad,	402	17%
L	Fish, tuna, fresh, bluefin, cooked, dry heat,	50	2%
L	Fish, tuna, fresh, bluefin, raw,	39	2%
L	Fish, tuna, fresh, skipjack, raw,	37	2%
L	Fish, tuna, fresh, yellowfin, raw,	45	2%
M	Fish, tuna, light, canned in oil, drained solids,	416	18%
L	Fish, tuna, light, canned in oil, without salt, drained solids,	50	2%
M	Fish, tuna, light, canned in water, drained solids,	247	11%
L	Fish, tuna, light, canned in water, without salt, drained solids,	50	2%
L	Fish, tuna, skipjack, fresh, cooked, dry heat,	47	2%
M	Fish, tuna, white, canned in oil, drained solids,	396	17%
L	Fish, tuna, white, canned in oil, without salt, drained solids,	50	2%
M	Fish, tuna, white, canned in water, drained solids,	377	16%
L	Fish, tuna, white, canned in water, without salt, drained solids,	50	2%
L	Fish, tuna, yellowfin, fresh, cooked, dry heat,	54	2%
M	Fish, turbot, european, cooked, dry heat,	192	8%
M	Fish, turbot, european, raw,	150	7%
L	Fish, whitefish, mixed species, cooked, dry heat,	65	3%
L	Fish, whitefish, mixed species, raw,	51	2%
H	Fish, whitefish, mixed species, smoked,	1019	44%
M	Fish, whiting, mixed species, cooked, dry heat,	132	6%
L	Fish, whiting, mixed species, raw,	72	3%
L	Fish, wolffish, atlantic, cooked, dry heat,	109	5%
L	Fish, wolffish, atlantic, raw,	85	4%
L	Fish, yellowtail, mixed species, cooked, dry heat,	50	2%
L	Fish, yellowtail, mixed species, raw,	39	2%

M	Flan, caramel custard, dry mix,	432	19%
H	Frankfurter, beef, heated,	852	37%
H	Frankfurter, beef, low fat,	744	32%
H	Frankfurter, beef, unheated,	992	43%
H	Frankfurter, chicken,	1027	45%
M	Frankfurter, low sodium,	311	14%
H	Frankfurter, meat and poultry, cooked, boiled,	914	40%
H	Frankfurter, meat and poultry, cooked, grilled,	1079	47%
H	Frankfurter, meat and poultry, low fat,	983	43%
H	Frankfurter, meat and poultry, unheated,	976	42%
H	Frankfurter, meat,	1090	47%
H	Frankfurter, meat, heated,	1013	44%
M	Frankfurter, meatless,	471	20%
H	Frankfurter, turkey,	911	40%
H	French toast, frozen, ready-to-heat,	495	22%
H	French toast, prepared from recipe, made with low fat (2%) milk,	479	21%
M	Frijoles rojos volteados (refried beans, red, canned),	375	16%
L	Frog legs, raw,	58	3%
L	Frostings, chocolate, creamy, dry mix,	76	3%
L	Frostings, chocolate, creamy, dry mix, prepared with butter,	124	5%
M	Frostings, chocolate, creamy, dry mix, prepared with margarine,	163	7%
M	Frostings, chocolate, creamy, ready-to-eat,	183	8%
M	Frostings, coconut-nut, ready-to-eat,	160	7%
M	Frostings, cream cheese-flavor, ready-to-eat,	191	8%
L	Frostings, vanilla, creamy, dry mix, prepared with margarine,	114	5%
M	Frostings, vanilla, creamy, ready-to-eat,	184	8%
M	Frostings, white, fluffy, dry mix,	234	10%
M	Frostings, white, fluffy, dry mix, prepared with water,	156	7%
L	Frozen novelties, fruit and juice bars,	0	0%
L	Frozen novelties, ice cream type, chocolate or caramel covered, with nuts,	92	4%
L	Frozen novelties, ice cream type, vanilla ice cream, light, no sugar added, chocolate coated,	104	5%

L	Frozen novelties, ice type, fruit, no sugar added,	0	0%
L	Frozen novelties, ice type, italian, restaurant-prepared,	0	0%
L	Frozen novelties, juice type, juice with cream,	42	2%
M	Frozen novelties, klondike, slim-a-bear chocolate cone,	159	7%
L	Frozen novelties, klondike, slim-a-bear fudge bar, 98% fat free, no sugar added,	120	5%
M	Frozen novelties, klondike, slim-a-bear vanilla sandwich,	191	8%
L	Frozen yogurts, chocolate,	63	3%
L	Frozen yogurts, chocolate, nonfat milk, sweetened without sugar,	81	4%
L	Frozen yogurts, chocolate, soft-serve,	98	4%
L	Frozen yogurts, flavors other than chocolate,	63	3%
L	Frozen yogurts, vanilla, soft-serve,	87	4%
L	Fruit cocktail, (peach and pineapple and pear and grape and cherry), canned, extra light syrup, solids and liquids,	0	0%
L	Fruit cocktail, (peach and pineapple and pear and grape and cherry), canned, juice pack, solids and liquids,	0	0%
L	Fruit cocktail, (peach and pineapple and pear and grape and cherry), canned, water pack, solids and liquids,	0	0%
L	Fruit flavored drink containing less than 3% fruit juice, with high vitamin c,	36	2%
L	Fruit flavored drink, less than 3% juice, not fortified with vitamin c,	36	2%
L	Fruit juice drink, greater than 3% fruit juice, high vitamin c and added thiamin,	61	3%
L	Fruit juice drink, reduced sugar, with vitamin e added,	0	0%
L	Fruit punch drink, frozen concentrate, prepared with water,	0	0%
L	Fruit punch drink, with added nutrients, canned,	38	2%
L	Fruit punch juice drink, frozen concentrate, prepared with water,	0	0%

L	Fruit salad, (peach and pear and apricot and pineapple and cherry), canned, extra heavy syrup, solids and liquids,	0	0%
L	Fruit salad, (peach and pear and apricot and pineapple and cherry), canned, juice pack, solids and liquids,	0	0%
L	Fruit salad, (peach and pear and apricot and pineapple and cherry), canned, water pack, solids and liquids,	0	0%
L	Fruit salad, (pineapple and papaya and banana and guava), tropical, canned, heavy syrup, solids and liquids,	0	0%
L	Fruit syrup,	0	0%
M	Fruit-flavored drink, dry powdered mix, low calorie, with aspartame,	404	18%
M	Frybread, made with lard (navajo),	329	14%
L	Game meat , bison, ground, raw,	66	3%
L	Game meat , bison, top sirloin, separable lean only, 1\ steak, cooked, broiled,	53	2%
L	Game meat, antelope, cooked, roasted,	54	2%
L	Game meat, antelope, raw,	51	2%
L	Game meat, bear, cooked, simmered,	71	3%
L	Game meat, beaver, cooked, roasted,	59	3%
L	Game meat, beaver, raw,	51	2%
L	Game meat, beefalo, composite of cuts, cooked, roasted,	82	4%
L	Game meat, beefalo, composite of cuts, raw,	78	3%
L	Game meat, bison, chuck, shoulder clod, separable lean only, cooked, braised,	57	2%
L	Game meat, bison, chuck, shoulder clod, separable lean only, raw,	62	3%
L	Game meat, bison, ground, cooked, pan-broiled,	73	3%
L	Game meat, bison, ribeye, separable lean only, 1\ steak, cooked, broiled,	52	2%
L	Game meat, bison, ribeye, separable lean only, trimmed to 0\ fat, raw,	48	2%
L	Game meat, bison, separable lean only, cooked, roasted,	57	2%
L	Game meat, bison, separable lean only, raw,	54	2%

L	Game meat, bison, shoulder clod, separable lean only, trimmed to 0\ fat, raw,	59	3%
L	Game meat, bison, top round, separable lean only, 1\ steak, cooked, broiled,	41	2%
L	Game meat, bison, top round, separable lean only, 1\ steak, raw,	47	2%
L	Game meat, bison, top sirloin, separable lean only, trimmed to 0\ fat, raw,	51	2%
L	Game meat, boar, wild, cooked, roasted,	60	3%
L	Game meat, buffalo, water, cooked, roasted,	56	2%
L	Game meat, buffalo, water, raw,	53	2%
L	Game meat, caribou, cooked, roasted,	60	3%
L	Game meat, caribou, raw,	57	2%
L	Game meat, deer, cooked, roasted,	54	2%
L	Game meat, deer, ground, cooked, pan-broiled,	78	3%
L	Game meat, deer, ground, raw,	75	3%
L	Game meat, deer, loin, separable lean only, 1\ steak, cooked, broiled,	57	2%
L	Game meat, deer, raw,	51	2%
L	Game meat, deer, shoulder clod, separable lean only, cooked, braised,	52	2%
L	Game meat, deer, tenderloin, separable lean only, cooked, broiled,	57	2%
L	Game meat, deer, top round, separable lean only, 1\ steak, cooked, broiled,	45	2%
L	Game meat, elk, cooked, roasted,	61	3%
L	Game meat, elk, ground, cooked, pan-broiled,	85	4%
L	Game meat, elk, ground, raw,	79	3%
L	Game meat, elk, loin, separable lean only, cooked, broiled,	54	2%
L	Game meat, elk, raw,	58	3%
L	Game meat, elk, round, separable lean only, cooked, broiled,	51	2%
L	Game meat, elk, tenderloin, separable lean only, cooked, broiled,	50	2%
L	Game meat, goat, cooked, roasted,	86	4%
L	Game meat, horse, cooked, roasted,	55	2%
L	Game meat, horse, raw,	53	2%
L	Game meat, moose, cooked, roasted,	69	3%

L	Game meat, moose, raw,	65	3%
L	Game meat, muskrat, cooked, roasted,	95	4%
L	Game meat, muskrat, raw,	82	4%
L	Game meat, opossum, cooked, roasted,	58	3%
L	Game meat, rabbit, domesticated, composite of cuts, cooked, roasted,	47	2%
L	Game meat, rabbit, domesticated, composite of cuts, cooked, stewed,	37	2%
L	Game meat, rabbit, domesticated, composite of cuts, raw,	41	2%
L	Game meat, rabbit, wild, cooked, stewed,	45	2%
L	Game meat, rabbit, wild, raw,	50	2%
L	Game meat, raccoon, cooked, roasted,	79	3%
L	Game meat, squirrel, cooked, roasted,	119	5%
L	Game meat, squirrel, raw,	103	4%
H	Garlic bread, frozen,	544	24%
M	Gelatin desserts, dry mix,	466	20%
L	Gelatin desserts, dry mix, prepared with water,	75	3%
H	Gelatin desserts, dry mix, reduced calorie, with aspartame,	862	37%
V.H	Gelatin desserts, dry mix, reduced calorie, with aspartame, added phosphorus, potassium, sodium, vitamin c,	2751	120%
M	Gelatin desserts, dry mix, reduced calorie, with aspartame, no added sodium,	158	7%
L	Gelatin desserts, dry mix, reduced calorie, with aspartame, prepared with water,	48	2%
H	Gelatin desserts, dry mix, with added ascorbic acid, sodium-citrate and salt,	491	21%
M	Gelatins, dry powder, unsweetened,	196	9%
L	Goat, raw,	82	4%
M	Goji berries, dried,	298	13%
L	Goose, domesticated, meat and skin, cooked, roasted,	70	3%
L	Goose, domesticated, meat and skin, raw,	73	3%
L	Goose, domesticated, meat only, cooked, roasted,	76	3%
L	Goose, domesticated, meat only, raw,	87	4%
M	Goose, liver, raw,	140	6%

L	Gooseberries, canned, light syrup pack, solids and liquids,	0	0%
L	Gooseberries, raw,	0	0%
M	Gourd, dishcloth (towelgourd), cooked, boiled, drained, with salt,	257	11%
L	Gourd, dishcloth (towelgourd), raw,	0	0%
M	Gourd, white-flowered (calabash), cooked, boiled, drained, with salt,	238	10%
L	Gourd, white-flowered (calabash), cooked, boiled, drained, without salt,	0	0%
L	Gourd, white-flowered (calabash), raw,	0	0%
M	Granola bar, soft, milk chocolate coated, peanut butter,	193	8%
L	Grape juice, canned or bottled, unsweetened, with added ascorbic acid and calcium,	0	0%
L	Grape juice, canned or bottled, unsweetened, with added ascorbic acid,	0	0%
L	Grape juice, canned or bottled, unsweetened, without added ascorbic acid,	0	0%
V.H	Grape leaves, canned,	2853	124%
L	Grapefruit juice, pink or red, with added calcium,	0	0%
L	Grapefruit juice, pink, raw,	0	0%
L	Grapefruit juice, white, bottled, unsweetened, ocean spray,	0	0%
L	Grapefruit juice, white, canned or bottled, unsweetened,	0	0%
L	Grapefruit juice, white, canned, sweetened,	0	0%
L	Grapefruit juice, white, frozen concentrate, unsweetened, diluted with 3 volume water,	0	0%
L	Grapefruit juice, white, frozen concentrate, unsweetened, undiluted,	0	0%
L	Grapefruit juice, white, raw,	0	0%
L	Grapefruit, raw, pink and red and white, all areas,	0	0%
L	Grapefruit, raw, pink and red, all areas,	0	0%
L	Grapefruit, raw, pink and red, california and arizona,	0	0%
L	Grapefruit, raw, pink and red, florida,	0	0%
L	Grapefruit, raw, white, all areas,	0	0%

L	Grapefruit, raw, white, california,	0	0%
L	Grapefruit, raw, white, florida,	0	0%
L	Grapefruit, sections, canned, light syrup pack, solids and liquids,	0	0%
L	Grapefruit, sections, canned, water pack, solids and liquids,	0	0%
L	Grapes, american type (slip skin), raw,	0	0%
L	Grapes, canned, thompson seedless, heavy syrup pack, solids and liquids,	0	0%
L	Grapes, muscadine, raw,	0	0%
L	Grapes, red or green (european type, such as thompson seedless), raw,	0	0%
H	Gravy, au jus, canned,	478	21%
V.H	Gravy, au jus, dry,	11588	504%
H	Gravy, beef, canned, ready-to-serve,	560	24%
V.H	Gravy, brown instant, dry,	5053	220%
V.H	Gravy, brown, dry,	4843	211%
V.H	Gravy, instant beef, dry,	5203	226%
V.H	Gravy, instant turkey, dry,	4090	178%
H	Gravy, mushroom, canned,	570	25%
V.H	Gravy, mushroom, dry, powder,	6580	286%
V.H	Gravy, onion, dry, mix,	4186	182%
H	Gravy, turkey, canned, ready-to-serve,	577	25%
V.H	Gravy, turkey, dry,	4392	191%
V.H	Gravy, unspecified type, dry,	5730	249%
L	Ground turkey, 85% lean, 15% fat, pan-broiled crumbles,	85	4%
L	Ground turkey, 85% lean, 15% fat, patties, broiled,	81	4%
L	Ground turkey, 85% lean, 15% fat, raw,	54	2%
L	Ground turkey, 93% lean, 7% fat, pan-broiled crumbles,	90	4%
L	Ground turkey, 93% lean, 7% fat, patties, broiled,	91	4%
L	Ground turkey, 93% lean, 7% fat, raw,	69	3%
L	Ground turkey, cooked,	78	3%
L	Ground turkey, fat free, pan-broiled crumbles,	61	3%
L	Ground turkey, fat free, patties, broiled,	59	3%
L	Ground turkey, fat free, raw,	51	2%
L	Ground turkey, raw,	58	3%

L	Guava sauce, cooked,	0	0%
L	Guavas, common, raw,	0	0%
L	Guavas, strawberry, raw,	37	2%
L	Guinca hcn, meat and skin, raw,	67	3%
L	Guinea hen, meat only, raw,	69	3%
L	Gums, seed gums (includes locust bean, guar),	125	5%
L	Hazelnuts, beaked (northern plains indians),	0	0%
M	Hominy, canned, white,	345	15%
M	Hominy, canned, yellow,	345	15%
H	Honey roll sausage, beef,	1322	57%
L	Honey,	0	0%
L	Horchata, dry mix, unprepared, variety of brands, all with morro seeds,	0	0%
L	Horned melon (kiwano),	0	0%
M	Horseradish, prepared,	420	18%
M	Hummus, commercial,	379	16%
M	Hummus, home prepared,	242	11%
H	Hush puppies, prepared from recipe,	668	29%
M	Hyacinth beans, mature seeds, cooked, boiled, with salt,	243	11%
M	Hyacinth-beans, immature seeds, cooked, boiled, drained, with salt,	238	10%
L	Hyacinth-beans, immature seeds, cooked, boiled, drained, without salt,	0	0%
L	Hyacinth-beans, immature seeds, raw,	0	0%
L	Ice cream bar, stick or nugget, with crunch coating,	84	4%
L	Ice cream cone, chocolate covered, with nuts, flavors other than chocolate,	94	4%
M	Ice cream cones, cake or wafer-type,	256	11%
M	Ice cream cones, sugar, rolled-type,	298	13%
M	Ice cream cookie sandwich,	162	7%
M	Ice cream sandwich,	129	6%
M	Ice cream sandwich, made with light ice cream, vanilla,	146	6%
M	Ice cream sandwich, vanilla, light, no sugar added,	164	7%
L	Ice cream, bar or stick, chocolate covered,	68	3%
L	Ice cream, light, soft serve, chocolate,	64	3%

L	Ice cream, soft serve, chocolate,	61	3%
L	Ice creams, chocolate,	76	3%
L	Ice creams, chocolate, light,	71	3%
L	Ice creams, chocolate, light, no sugar added,	75	3%
L	Ice creams, chocolate, rich,	57	2%
L	Ice creams, french vanilla, soft-serve,	61	3%
L	Ice creams, regular, low carbohydrate, chocolate,	76	3%
L	Ice creams, regular, low carbohydrate, vanilla,	48	2%
L	Ice creams, strawberry,	60	3%
L	Ice creams, vanilla,	80	3%
L	Ice creams, vanilla, fat free,	97	4%
L	Ice creams, vanilla, light,	74	3%
L	Ice creams, vanilla, light, no sugar added,	96	4%
L	Ice creams, vanilla, light, soft-serve,	70	3%
L	Ice creams, vanilla, rich,	61	3%
H	Imitation cheese, american or cheddar, low cholesterol,	670	29%
L	Incaparina, dry mix (corn and soy flours), unprepared,	0	0%
M	Instant breakfast powder, chocolate, not reconstituted,	385	17%
H	Instant breakfast powder, chocolate, sugar-free, not reconstituted,	717	31%
L	Jams and preserves, apricot,	40	2%
L	Jams and preserves, no sugar (with sodium saccharin), any flavor,	0	0%
L	Jellies, no sugar (with sodium saccharin), any flavors,	0	0%
L	Jellies, reduced sugar, home preserved,	0	0%
V.H	Jellyfish, dried, salted,	9690	421%
L	Juice, apple, grape and pear blend, with added ascorbic acid and calcium,	0	0%
M	Jute, potherb, cooked, boiled, drained, with salt,	247	11%
M	Kale, cooked, boiled, drained, with salt,	259	11%
M	Kale, frozen, cooked, boiled, drained, with salt,	251	11%
L	Kale, raw,	38	2%

M	Kale, scotch, cooked, boiled, drained, with salt,	281	12%
L	Kale, scotch, cooked, boiled, drained, without salt,	45	2%
L	Kale, scotch, raw,	70	3%
L	Lamb, ground, cooked, broiled,	81	4%
L	Lamb, ground, raw,	59	3%
L	Lamb, new zealand, imported, brains, cooked, soaked and fried,	101	4%
L	Lamb, new zealand, imported, brains, raw,	117	5%
M	Lamb, variety meats and by-products, brain, cooked, braised,	134	6%
M	Lamb, variety meats and by-products, brain, cooked, pan-fried,	157	7%
L	Lamb, variety meats and by-products, brain, raw,	112	5%
L	Lamb, variety meats and by-products, heart, cooked, braised,	63	3%
L	Lamb, variety meats and by-products, heart, raw,	89	4%
M	Lamb, variety meats and by-products, kidneys, cooked, braised,	151	7%
M	Lamb, variety meats and by-products, kidneys, raw,	156	7%
L	Lamb, variety meats and by-products, liver, cooked, braised,	56	2%
L	Lamb, variety meats and by-products, liver, cooked, pan-fried,	124	5%
L	Lamb, variety meats and by-products, liver, raw,	70	3%
L	Lamb, variety meats and by-products, lungs, cooked, braised,	84	4%
M	Lamb, variety meats and by-products, lungs, raw,	157	7%
L	Lamb, variety meats and by-products, mechanically separated, raw,	59	3%
L	Lamb, variety meats and by-products, pancreas, cooked, braised,	52	2%
L	Lamb, variety meats and by-products, pancreas, raw,	75	3%

L	Lamb, variety meats and by-products, spleen, cooked, braised,	58	3%
L	Lamb, variety meats and by-products, spleen, raw,	84	4%
L	Lamb, variety meats and by-products, tongue, cooked, braised,	67	3%
L	Lamb, variety meats and by-products, tongue, raw,	78	3%
M	Lambsquarters, cooked, boiled, drained, with salt,	265	12%
L	Lambsquarters, steamed (northern plains indians),	0	0%
L	Lard,	0	0%
M	Lasagna with meat & sauce, frozen entree,	347	15%
M	Lasagna with meat & sauce, low-fat, frozen entree,	181	8%
M	Lasagna with meat sauce, frozen, prepared,	373	16%
M	Lasagna, cheese, frozen, prepared,	284	12%
M	Lasagna, cheese, frozen, unprepared,	312	14%
M	Lasagna, vegetable, frozen, baked,	445	19%
H	Lean pockets, meatballs & mozzarella,	557	24%
V.H	Leavening agents, baking powder, double-acting, sodium aluminum sulfate,	10600	461%
V.H	Leavening agents, baking powder, double-acting, straight phosphate,	7893	343%
L	Leavening agents, baking powder, low-sodium,	90	4%
V.H	Leavening agents, baking soda,	27360	1190%
L	Leavening agents, cream of tartar,	52	2%
L	Leavening agents, yeast, baker's, active dry,	51	2%
H	Lebanon bologna, beef,	1374	60%
M	Leeks, (bulb and lower leaf-portion), cooked, boiled, drained, with salt,	246	11%
L	Lemon juice, frozen, unsweetened, single strength,	0	0%
L	Lemon juice, raw,	0	0%
L	Lemonade fruit juice drink light, fortified with vitamin e and c,	0	0%
M	Lemonade-flavor drink, powder,	130	6%
L	Lemonade, frozen concentrate, pink,	0	0%

L	Lemonade, frozen concentrate, pink, prepared with water,	0	0%
L	Lemonade, frozen concentrate, white, prepared wlth water,	0	0%
L	Lemonade, powder,	51	2%
L	Lemons, raw, without peel,	0	0%
M	Lentils, mature seeds, cooked, boiled, with salt,	238	10%
L	Lentils, mature seeds, cooked, boiled, without salt,	0	0%
L	Lettuce, butterhead (includes boston and bibb types), raw,	0	0%
L	Light ice cream, soft serve, blended with cookie pieces,	75	3%
L	Light ice cream, soft serve, blended with milk chocolate candies,	54	2%
L	Lima beans, immature seeds, canned, no salt added, solids and liquids,	0	0%
M	Lima beans, immature seeds, canned, regular pack, solids and liquids,	252	11%
M	Lima beans, immature seeds, cooked, boiled, drained, with salt,	253	11%
M	Lima beans, immature seeds, frozen, baby, cooked, boiled, drained, with salt,	265	12%
L	Lima beans, immature seeds, frozen, baby, unprepared,	52	2%
M	Lima beans, immature seeds, frozen, fordhook, cooked, boiled, drained, with salt,	289	13%
L	Lima beans, immature seeds, frozen, fordhook, cooked, boiled, drained, without salt,	69	3%
L	Lima beans, immature seeds, frozen, fordhook, unprepared,	58	3%
M	Lima beans, large, mature seeds, canned,	336	15%
M	Lima beans, large, mature seeds, cooked, boiled, with salt,	238	10%
L	Lima beans, large, mature seeds, cooked, boiled, without salt,	0	0%
M	Lima beans, thin seeded (baby), mature seeds, cooked, boiled, with salt,	239	10%

L	Lima beans, thin seeded (baby), mature seeds, cooked, boiled, without salt,	0	0%
L	Lime juice, raw,	0	0%
L	Limeade, frozen concentrate, prepared with water,	0	0%
L	Limes, raw,	0	0%
L	Litchis, dried,	0	0%
L	Litchis, raw,	0	0%
L	Longans, dried,	48	2%
L	Longans, raw,	0	0%
L	Loquats, raw,	0	0%
M	Lotus root, cooked, boiled, drained, with salt,	281	12%
L	Lotus root, cooked, boiled, drained, without salt,	45	2%
L	Lotus root, raw,	40	2%
H	Luncheon slices, meatless,	711	31%
M	Lupins, mature seeds, cooked, boiled, with salt,	240	10%
L	Lupins, mature seeds, cooked, boiled, without salt,	0	0%
H	Macaroni and cheese dinner with dry sauce mix, boxed, uncooked,	680	30%
M	Macaroni and cheese, box mix with cheese sauce, prepared,	460	20%
H	Macaroni and cheese, box mix with cheese sauce, unprepared,	766	33%
M	Macaroni and cheese, canned entree,	302	13%
M	Macaroni and cheese, canned, microwavable,	335	15%
M	Macaroni and cheese, dry mix, prepared with 2% milk and 80% stick margarine from dry mix,	338	15%
M	Macaroni and cheese, frozen entree,	290	13%
H	Macaroni or noodles with cheese, made from reduced fat packaged mix, unprepared,	867	38%
H	Macaroni or noodles with cheese, microwaveable, unprepared,	902	39%
L	Macaroni, vegetable, enriched, dry,	43	2%
L	Malabar spinach, cooked,	55	2%
L	Malt liquor beverage,	0	0%
M	Malted drink mix, chocolate, powder,	190	8%

L	Malted drink mix, chocolate, powder, prepared with whole milk,	60	3%
L	Malted drink mix, chocolate, with added nutrients, powder, prepared with whole milk,	87	4%
M	Malted drink mix, natural, powder, dairy based.,	405	18%
L	Malted drink mix, natural, powder, prepared with whole milk,	79	3%
L	Malted drink mix, natural, with added nutrients, powder, prepared with whole milk,	72	3%
L	Mango nectar, canned,	0	0%
L	Mangos, raw,	0	0%
L	Maraschino cherries, canned, drained,	0	0%
H	Margarine spread, approximately 48% fat, tub,	646	28%
H	Margarine-like shortening, industrial, soy (partially hydrogenated), cottonseed, and soy, principal use flaky pastries,	864	38%
H	Margarine-like spread with yogurt, 70% fat, stick, with salt,	590	26%
H	Margarine-like spread with yogurt, approximately 40% fat, tub, with salt,	630	27%
H	Margarine-like vegetable-oil spread, stick\/tub\/bottle, 60% fat, with added vitamin d,	785	34%
H	Margarine-like, margarine-butter blend, soybean oil and butter,	719	31%
H	Margarine-like, vegetable oil spread, 20% fat, with salt,	733	32%
L	Margarine-like, vegetable oil spread, 20% fat, without salt,	0	0%
H	Margarine-like, vegetable oil spread, 60% fat, stick, with salt,	785	34%
H	Margarine-like, vegetable oil spread, 60% fat, stick, with salt, with added vitamin d,	785	34%
H	Margarine-like, vegetable oil spread, 60% fat, stick\/tub\/bottle, with salt,	700	30%
L	Margarine-like, vegetable oil spread, 60% fat, stick\/tub\/bottle, without salt,	0	0%

L	Margarine-like, vegetable oil spread, 60% fat, stick\/tub\/bottle, without salt, with added vitamin d,	0	0%
H	Margarine-like, vegetable oil spread, 60% fat, tub, with salt,	615	27%
H	Margarine-like, vegetable oil spread, 60% fat, tub, with salt, with added vitamin d,	785	34%
H	Margarine-like, vegetable oil spread, approximately 37% fat, unspecified oils, with salt, with added vitamin d,	589	26%
H	Margarine-like, vegetable oil spread, fat free, liquid, with salt,	833	36%
H	Margarine-like, vegetable oil spread, fat-free, tub,	580	25%
H	Margarine-like, vegetable oil spread, stick or tub, sweetened,	542	24%
H	Margarine-like, vegetable oil spread, unspecified oils, approximately 37% fat, with salt,	589	26%
H	Margarine-like, vegetable oil-butter spread, reduced calorie, tub, with salt,	607	26%
H	Margarine-like, vegetable oil-butter spread, tub, with salt,	786	34%
H	Margarine, 80% fat, stick, includes regular and hydrogenated corn and soybean oils,	654	28%
H	Margarine, 80% fat, tub, canola harvest soft spread (canola, palm and palm kernel oils),	714	31%
H	Margarine, industrial, non-dairy, cottonseed, soy oil (partially hydrogenated), for flaky pastries,	879	38%
H	Margarine, industrial, soy and partially hydrogenated soy oil, use for baking, sauces and candy,	886	39%
H	Margarine, margarine-like vegetable oil spread, 67-70% fat, tub,	536	23%
H	Margarine, margarine-type vegetable oil spread, 70% fat, soybean and partially hydrogenated soybean, stick,	700	30%
H	Margarine, regular, 80% fat, composite, stick, with salt,	751	33%

H	Margarine, regular, 80% fat, composite, stick, with salt, with added vitamin d,	751	33%
L	Margarine, regular, 80% fat, composite, stick, without salt,	0	0%
L	Margarine, regular, 80% fat, composite, stick, without salt, with added vitamin d,	0	0%
H	Margarine, regular, 80% fat, composite, tub, with salt,	657	29%
H	Margarine, regular, 80% fat, composite, tub, with salt, with added vitamin d,	657	29%
H	Margarine, regular, hard, soybean (hydrogenated),	943	41%
L	Marmalade, orange,	56	2%
L	Meal supplement drink, canned, peanut flavor,	54	2%
H	Meat drippings (lard, beef tallow, mutton tallow),	545	24%
H	Meatballs, frozen, italian style,	666	29%
H	Meatballs, meatless,	550	24%
M	Milk and cereal bar,	319	14%
L	Milk dessert bar, frozen, made from lowfat milk,	92	4%
L	Milk dessert, frozen, milk-fat free, chocolate,	97	4%
L	Milk reduced fat, flavored and sweetened, ready-to-drink, added calcium, vitamin a and vitamin d,	49	2%
L	Milk shakes, thick chocolate,	111	5%
L	Milk shakes, thick vanilla,	95	4%
L	Milk substitutes, fluid, with lauric acid oil,	78	3%
H	Milk, buttermilk, dried,	517	22%
M	Milk, buttermilk, fluid, cultured, lowfat,	190	8%
L	Milk, buttermilk, fluid, cultured, reduced fat,	105	5%
L	Milk, buttermilk, fluid, whole,	105	5%
M	Milk, canned, condensed, sweetened,	127	6%
L	Milk, canned, evaporated, nonfat, with added vitamin a and vitamin d,	115	5%
L	Milk, canned, evaporated, with added vitamin a,	106	5%
L	Milk, canned, evaporated, with added vitamin d and without added vitamin a,	106	5%

L	Milk, canned, evaporated, without added vitamin a and vitamin d,	106	5%
L	Milk, chocolate hot cocoa, homemade,	44	2%
L	Milk, chocolate, fluid, commercial, reduced fat, with added calcium,	66	3%
L	Milk, chocolate, fluid, commercial, reduced fat, with added vitamin a and vitamin d,	66	3%
L	Milk, chocolate, fluid, commercial, whole, with added vitamin a and vitamin d,	60	3%
L	Milk, chocolate, lowfat, with added vitamin a and vitamin d,	65	3%
H	Milk, dry, nonfat, calcium reduced,	2280	99%
H	Milk, dry, nonfat, instant, with added vitamin a and vitamin d,	549	24%
H	Milk, dry, nonfat, instant, without added vitamin a and vitamin d,	549	24%
H	Milk, dry, nonfat, regular, with added vitamin a and vitamin d,	535	23%
H	Milk, dry, nonfat, regular, without added vitamin a and vitamin d,	535	23%
M	Milk, dry, whole, with added vitamin d,	371	16%
M	Milk, dry, whole, without added vitamin d,	371	16%
L	Milk, evaporated, 2% fat, with added vitamin a and vitamin d,	100	4%
L	Milk, filled, fluid, with blend of hydrogenated vegetable oils,	57	2%
L	Milk, filled, fluid, with lauric acid oil,	57	2%
L	Milk, fluid, 1% fat, without added vitamin a and vitamin d,	44	2%
L	Milk, fluid, nonfat, calcium fortified (fat free or skim),	52	2%
L	Milk, goat, fluid, with added vitamin d,	50	2%
L	Milk, imitation, non-soy,	55	2%
L	Milk, indian buffalo, fluid,	52	2%
L	Milk, low sodium, fluid,	0	0%
L	Milk, lowfat, fluid, 1% milkfat, protein fortified, with added vitamin a and vitamin d,	58	3%
L	Milk, lowfat, fluid, 1% milkfat, with added nonfat milk solids, vitamin a and vitamin d,	52	2%

L	Milk, lowfat, fluid, 1% milkfat, with added vitamin a and vitamin d,	44	2%
L	Milk, nonfat, fluid, protein fortified, with added vitamin a and vitamin d (fat free and skim),	59	3%
L	Milk, nonfat, fluid, with added nonfat milk solids, vitamin a and vitamin d (fat free or skim),	53	2%
L	Milk, nonfat, fluid, with added vitamin a and vitamin d (fat free or skim),	42	2%
L	Milk, nonfat, fluid, without added vitamin a and vitamin d (fat free or skim),	42	2%
L	Milk, producer, fluid, 3.7% milkfat,	49	2%
L	Milk, reduced fat, fluid, 2% milkfat, protein fortified, with added vitamin a and vitamin d,	59	3%
L	Milk, reduced fat, fluid, 2% milkfat, with added nonfat milk solids and vitamin a and vitamin d,	52	2%
L	Milk, reduced fat, fluid, 2% milkfat, with added nonfat milk solids, without added vitamin a,	59	3%
L	Milk, reduced fat, fluid, 2% milkfat, with added vitamin a and vitamin d,	47	2%
L	Milk, reduced fat, fluid, 2% milkfat, without added vitamin a and vitamin d,	47	2%
L	Milk, sheep, fluid,	44	2%
L	Milk, whole, 3.25% milkfat, with added vitamin d,	43	2%
L	Milk, whole, 3.25% milkfat, without added vitamin a and vitamin d,	43	2%
H	Milkshake mix, dry, not chocolate,	780	34%
L	Millet flour,	0	0%
L	Millet, cooked,	0	0%
L	Millet, puffed,	0	0%
L	Millet, raw,	0	0%
V.H	Miso,	3728	162%
L	Molasses,	37	2%
H	Mollusks, abalone, mixed species, cooked, fried,	591	26%
M	Mollusks, abalone, mixed species, raw,	301	13%
L	Mollusks, clam, mixed species, canned, drained solids,	112	5%

M	Mollusks, clam, mixed species, canned, liquid,	215	9%
M	Mollusks, clam, mixed species, cooked, breaded and fried,	364	16%
H	Mollusks, clam, mixed species, cooked, moist heat,	1202	52%
H	Mollusks, clam, mixed species, raw,	601	26%
M	Mollusks, conch, baked or broiled,	153	7%
H	Mollusks, cuttlefish, mixed species, cooked, moist heat,	744	32%
M	Mollusks, cuttlefish, mixed species, raw,	372	16%
M	Mollusks, mussel, blue, cooked, moist heat,	369	16%
M	Mollusks, mussel, blue, raw,	286	12%
M	Mollusks, octopus, common, cooked, moist heat,	460	20%
M	Mollusks, octopus, common, raw,	230	10%
L	Mollusks, oyster, eastern, canned,	112	5%
M	Mollusks, oyster, eastern, cooked, breaded and fried,	417	18%
M	Mollusks, oyster, eastern, farmed, cooked, dry heat,	163	7%
M	Mollusks, oyster, eastern, farmed, raw,	178	8%
M	Mollusks, oyster, eastern, wild, cooked, dry heat,	132	6%
M	Mollusks, oyster, eastern, wild, cooked, moist heat,	166	7%
L	Mollusks, oyster, eastern, wild, raw,	85	4%
M	Mollusks, oyster, pacific, cooked, moist heat,	212	9%
L	Mollusks, oyster, pacific, raw,	106	5%
H	Mollusks, scallop, (bay and sea), cooked, steamed,	667	29%
M	Mollusks, scallop, mixed species, cooked, breaded and fried,	464	20%
H	Mollusks, scallop, mixed species, imitation, made from surimi,	795	35%
M	Mollusks, scallop, mixed species, raw,	392	17%
L	Mollusks, snail, raw,	70	3%
M	Mollusks, squid, mixed species, cooked, fried,	306	13%
L	Mollusks, squid, mixed species, raw,	44	2%

M	Mollusks, whelk, unspecified, cooked, moist heat,	412	18%
M	Mollusks, whelk, unspecified, raw,	206	9%
M	Mountain yam, hawaii, cooked, steamed, with salt,	248	11%
M	Muffin, blueberry, commercially prepared, low-fat,	413	18%
M	Muffins, blueberry, commercially prepared (includes mini-muffins),	336	15%
H	Muffins, blueberry, dry mix,	479	21%
M	Muffins, blueberry, prepared from recipe, made with low fat (2%) milk,	441	19%
M	Muffins, blueberry, toaster-type,	417	18%
M	Muffins, blueberry, toaster-type, toasted,	444	19%
M	Muffins, corn, commercially prepared,	467	20%
H	Muffins, corn, dry mix, prepared,	795	35%
H	Muffins, corn, prepared from recipe, made with low fat (2%) milk,	585	25%
M	Muffins, corn, toaster-type,	430	19%
M	Muffins, oat bran,	393	17%
M	Muffins, plain, prepared from recipe, made with low fat (2%) milk,	467	20%
H	Muffins, wheat bran, dry mix,	700	30%
H	Muffins, wheat bran, toaster-type with raisins, toasted,	527	23%
M	Mung beans, mature seeds, cooked, boiled, with salt,	238	10%
L	Mung beans, mature seeds, cooked, boiled, without salt,	0	0%
M	Mung beans, mature seeds, sprouted, cooked, boiled, drained, with salt,	246	11%
M	Mungo beans, mature seeds, cooked, boiled, with salt,	243	11%
L	Mushroom, white, exposed to ultraviolet light, raw,	0	0%
M	Mushrooms, canned, drained solids,	425	18%
L	Mushrooms, enoki, raw,	0	0%
L	Mushrooms, maitake, raw,	0	0%
M	Mushrooms, shiitake, cooked, with salt,	240	10%
L	Mushrooms, shiitake, cooked, without salt,	0	0%

L	Mushrooms, shiitake, stir-fried,	0	0%
M	Mushrooms, straw, canned, drained solids,	384	17%
M	Mushrooms, white, cooked, boiled, drained, with salt,	238	10%
L	Mushrooms, white, cooked, boiled, drained, without salt,	0	0%
L	Mushrooms, white, raw,	0	0%
M	Mustard greens, cooked, boiled, drained, with salt,	252	11%
M	Mustard greens, frozen, cooked, boiled, drained, with salt,	261	11%
M	Mustard spinach, (tendergreen), cooked, boiled, drained, with salt,	250	11%
H	Mustard, prepared, yellow,	1104	48%
M	Mutton, cooked, roasted (navajo),	135	6%
L	Naranjilla (lulo) pulp, frozen, unsweetened,	0	0%
L	Nectarines, raw,	0	0%
M	New zealand spinach, cooked, boiled, drained, with salt,	343	15%
L	New zealand spinach, cooked, boiled, drained, without salt,	107	5%
M	New zealand spinach, raw,	130	6%
H	Noodles, chinese, chow mein,	1174	51%
M	Noodles, egg, cooked, enriched, with added salt,	165	7%
M	Noodles, egg, cooked, unenriched, with added salt,	165	7%
L	Noodles, egg, enriched, cooked,	0	0%
L	Noodles, egg, spinach, enriched, dry,	72	3%
L	Noodles, egg, unenriched, cooked, without added salt,	0	0%
M	Noodles, flat, crunchy, chinese restaurant,	378	16%
L	Noodles, japanese, soba, cooked,	60	3%
H	Noodles, japanese, soba, dry,	792	34%
M	Noodles, japanese, somen, cooked,	161	7%
H	Noodles, japanese, somen, dry,	1840	80%
H	Nutritional shake mix, high protein, powder,	1214	53%
L	Nutritional supplement for people with diabetes, liquid,	92	4%
L	Nuts, acorn flour, full fat,	0	0%

L	Nuts, acorns, dried,	0	0%
L	Nuts, acorns, raw,	0	0%
M	Nuts, almond butter, plain, with salt added,	227	10%
L	Nuts, almonds,	0	0%
H	Nuts, almonds, dry roasted, with salt added,	498	22%
L	Nuts, almonds, dry roasted, without salt added,	0	0%
M	Nuts, almonds, honey roasted, unblanched,	130	6%
M	Nuts, almonds, oil roasted, lightly salted,	143	6%
M	Nuts, almonds, oil roasted, with salt added,	339	15%
H	Nuts, almonds, oil roasted, with salt added, smoke flavor,	548	24%
L	Nuts, almonds, oil roasted, without salt added,	0	0%
L	Nuts, beechnuts, dried,	38	2%
L	Nuts, brazilnuts, dried, unblanched,	0	0%
L	Nuts, butternuts, dried,	0	0%
M	Nuts, cashew butter, plain, with salt added,	295	13%
H	Nuts, cashew nuts, dry roasted, with salt added,	640	28%
M	Nuts, cashew nuts, oil roasted, with salt added,	308	13%
L	Nuts, chestnuts, chinese, boiled and steamed,	0	0%
L	Nuts, chestnuts, chinese, dried,	0	0%
L	Nuts, chestnuts, chinese, raw,	0	0%
L	Nuts, chestnuts, chinese, roasted,	0	0%
L	Nuts, chestnuts, european, dried, peeled,	37	2%
L	Nuts, chestnuts, european, dried, unpeeled,	37	2%
L	Nuts, chestnuts, european, raw, peeled,	0	0%
L	Nuts, chestnuts, european, raw, unpeeled,	0	0%
L	Nuts, chestnuts, european, roasted,	0	0%
L	Nuts, chestnuts, japanese, boiled and steamed,	0	0%
L	Nuts, coconut cream, canned, sweetened,	36	2%
L	Nuts, coconut cream, raw (liquid expressed from grated meat),	0	0%
L	Nuts, coconut meat, dried (desiccated), creamed,	37	2%

L	Nuts, coconut meat, dried (desiccated), not sweetened,	37	2%
M	Nuts, coconut meat, dried (desiccated), sweetened, flaked, packaged,	285	12%
M	Nuts, coconut meat, dried (desiccated), sweetened, shredded,	262	11%
L	Nuts, coconut meat, dried (desiccated), toasted,	37	2%
L	Nuts, coconut water (liquid from coconuts),	105	5%
L	Nuts, formulated, wheat-based, all flavors except macadamia, without salt,	91	4%
H	Nuts, formulated, wheat-based, unflavored, with salt added,	505	22%
M	Nuts, ginkgo nuts, canned,	307	13%
L	Nuts, hazelnuts or filberts,	0	0%
L	Nuts, hazelnuts or filberts, blanched,	0	0%
L	Nuts, hazelnuts or filberts, dry roasted, without salt added,	0	0%
L	Nuts, hickorynuts, dried,	0	0%
M	Nuts, macadamia nuts, dry roasted, with salt added,	353	15%
L	Nuts, macadamia nuts, dry roasted, without salt added,	0	0%
L	Nuts, macadamia nuts, raw,	0	0%
M	Nuts, mixed nuts, dry roasted, with peanuts, with salt added,	345	15%
L	Nuts, mixed nuts, dry roasted, with peanuts, without salt added,	0	0%
M	Nuts, mixed nuts, oil roasted, with peanuts, lightly salted,	161	7%
M	Nuts, mixed nuts, oil roasted, with peanuts, with salt added,	273	12%
L	Nuts, mixed nuts, oil roasted, with peanuts, without salt added,	0	0%
M	Nuts, mixed nuts, oil roasted, without peanuts, lightly salted,	143	6%
M	Nuts, mixed nuts, oil roasted, without peanuts, with salt added,	306	13%
L	Nuts, pecans,	0	0%
M	Nuts, pecans, dry roasted, with salt added,	383	17%

L	Nuts, pecans, dry roasted, without salt added,	0	0%
M	Nuts, pecans, oil roasted, with salt added,	393	17%
L	Nuts, pecans, oil roasted, without salt added,	0	0%
L	Nuts, pilinuts, dried,	0	0%
L	Nuts, pine nuts, dried,	0	0%
L	Nuts, pine nuts, pinyon, dried,	72	3%
M	Nuts, pistachio nuts, dry roasted, with salt added,	428	19%
L	Nuts, pistachio nuts, raw,	0	0%
L	Nuts, walnuts, black, dried,	0	0%
H	Nuts, walnuts, dry roasted, with salt added,	643	28%
L	Nuts, walnuts, english,	0	0%
M	Nuts, walnuts, glazed,	446	19%
L	Oat bran, cooked,	0	0%
L	Oat bran, raw,	0	0%
L	Oats,	0	0%
L	Oheloberries, raw,	0	0%
L	Oil, almond,	0	0%
L	Oil, apricot kernel,	0	0%
L	Oil, avocado,	0	0%
L	Oil, babassu,	0	0%
L	Oil, canola,	0	0%
L	Oil, cocoa butter,	0	0%
L	Oil, coconut,	0	0%
L	Oil, corn and canola,	0	0%
L	Oil, corn, industrial and retail, all purpose salad or cooking,	0	0%
L	Oil, corn, peanut, and olive,	0	0%
L	Oil, cottonseed, salad or cooking,	0	0%
L	Oil, cupu assu,	0	0%
L	Oil, flaxseed, cold pressed,	0	0%
L	Oil, grapeseed,	0	0%
L	Oil, hazelnut,	0	0%
L	Oil, industrial, canola (partially hydrogenated) oil for deep fat frying,	0	0%
L	Oil, industrial, canola for salads, woks and light frying,	0	0%
L	Oil, industrial, canola with antifoaming agent, principal uses salads, woks and light frying,	0	0%

L	Oil, industrial, canola, high oleic,	0	0%
L	Oil, industrial, coconut, confection fat, typical basis for ice cream coatings,	0	0%
L	Oil, industrial, coconut, principal uses candy coatings, oil sprays, roasting nuts,	0	0%
L	Oil, industrial, cottonseed, fully hydrogenated,	0	0%
L	Oil, industrial, mid-oleic, sunflower,	0	0%
L	Oil, industrial, soy (partially hydrogenated), all purpose,	0	0%
L	Oil, industrial, soy (partially hydrogenated) and soy (winterized), pourable clear fry,	0	0%
L	Oil, industrial, soy (partially hydrogenated), palm, principal uses icings and fillings,	0	0%
L	Oil, industrial, soy (partially hydrogenated) and cottonseed, principal use as a tortilla shortening,	0	0%
L	Oil, industrial, soy (partially hydrogenated), multiuse for non-dairy butter flavor,	0	0%
L	Oil, industrial, soy (partially hydrogenated), principal uses popcorn and flavoring vegetables,	0	0%
L	Oil, industrial, soy, fully hydrogenated,	0	0%
L	Oil, industrial, soy, low linolenic,	0	0%
L	Oil, industrial, soy, refined, for woks and light frying,	0	0%
L	Oil, industrial, soy, ultra low linolenic,	0	0%
L	Oil, mustard,	0	0%
L	Oil, nutmeg butter,	0	0%
L	Oil, oat,	0	0%
L	Oil, olive, salad or cooking,	0	0%
L	Oil, palm,	0	0%
L	Oil, peanut, salad or cooking,	0	0%
L	Oil, poppyseed,	0	0%
L	Oil, rice bran,	0	0%
L	Oil, safflower, salad or cooking, high oleic (primary safflower oil of commerce),	0	0%
L	Oil, safflower, salad or cooking, linoleic, (over 70%),	0	0%
L	Oil, sesame, salad or cooking,	0	0%
L	Oil, sheanut,	0	0%

L	Oil, soybean lecithin,	0	0%
L	Oil, soybean, salad or cooking,	0	0%
L	Oil, soybean, salad or cooking, (partially hydrogenated) and cottonseed,	0	0%
L	Oil, soybean, salad or cooking, (partially hydrogenated),	0	0%
L	Oil, sunflower, high oleic (70% and over),	0	0%
L	Oil, sunflower, linoleic (less than 60%),	0	0%
L	Oil, sunflower, linoleic, (approx. 65%),	0	0%
L	Oil, sunflower, linoleic, (partially hydrogenated),	0	0%
L	Oil, teaseed,	0	0%
L	Oil, tomatoseed,	0	0%
L	Oil, ucuhuba butter,	0	0%
L	Oil, vegetable, natreon canola, high stability, non trans, high oleic (70%),	0	0%
L	Oil, walnut,	0	0%
L	Oil, wheat germ,	0	0%
M	Okra, cooked, boiled, drained, with salt,	241	10%
M	Okra, frozen, cooked, boiled, drained, with salt,	239	10%
L	Okra, frozen, cooked, boiled, drained, without salt,	0	0%
L	Okra, frozen, unprepared,	0	0%
M	Onion rings, breaded, par fried, frozen, prepared, heated in oven,	370	16%
M	Onion rings, breaded, par fried, frozen, unprepared,	246	11%
M	Onions, canned, solids and liquids,	371	16%
M	Onions, cooked, boiled, drained, with salt,	239	10%
L	Onions, cooked, boiled, drained, without salt,	0	0%
M	Onions, frozen, chopped, cooked, boiled, drained, with salt,	248	11%
M	Onions, frozen, whole, cooked, boiled, drained, with salt,	244	11%
L	Onions, raw,	0	0%
L	Orange and apricot juice drink, canned,	0	0%
L	Orange breakfast drink, ready-to-drink, with added nutrients,	54	2%
L	Orange drink, canned, with added vitamin c,	0	0%

L	Orange juice drink,	0	0%
L	Orange juice, canned, unsweetened,	0	0%
L	Orange juice, chilled, includes from concentrate,	0	0%
L	Orange juice, chilled, includes from concentrate, with added calcium and vitamin d,	0	0%
L	Orange juice, chilled, includes from concentrate, with added calcium and vitamins a, d, e,	0	0%
L	Orange juice, chilled, includes from concentrate, with added calcium,	0	0%
L	Orange juice, frozen concentrate, unsweetened, diluted with 3 volume water,	0	0%
L	Orange juice, frozen concentrate, unsweetened, diluted with 3 volume water, with added calcium,	0	0%
L	Orange juice, light, no pulp,	0	0%
L	Orange juice, raw,	0	0%
L	Orange peel, raw,	0	0%
L	Orange pineapple juice blend,	0	0%
L	Orange-flavor drink, breakfast type, low calorie, powder,	81	4%
L	Orange-flavor drink, breakfast type, powder, prepared with water,	0	0%
L	Orange-grapefruit juice, canned or bottled, unsweetened,	0	0%
L	Oranges, raw, all commercial varieties,	0	0%
L	Oranges, raw, california, valencias,	0	0%
L	Oranges, raw, florida,	0	0%
L	Oranges, raw, navels,	0	0%
L	Oranges, raw, with peel,	0	0%
L	Ostrich, fan, raw,	75	3%
L	Ostrich, ground, cooked, pan-broiled,	80	3%
L	Ostrich, ground, raw,	72	3%
L	Ostrich, inside leg, cooked,	83	4%
L	Ostrich, inside leg, raw,	72	3%
L	Ostrich, inside strip, cooked,	73	3%
L	Ostrich, inside strip, raw,	76	3%
L	Ostrich, outside leg, raw,	90	4%

L	Ostrich, outside strip, cooked,	72	3%
L	Ostrich, outside strip, raw,	70	3%
L	Ostrich, oyster, cooked,	81	4%
L	Ostrich, oyster, raw,	83	4%
L	Ostrich, round, raw,	72	3%
L	Ostrich, tenderloin, raw,	86	4%
L	Ostrich, tip trimmed, cooked,	80	3%
L	Ostrich, tip trimmed, raw,	67	3%
L	Ostrich, top loin, cooked,	77	3%
L	Ostrich, top loin, raw,	81	4%
L	Papaya nectar, canned,	0	0%
H	Parmesan cheese topping, fat free,	1150	50%
M	Parsley, freeze-dried,	391	17%
L	Parsley, fresh,	56	2%
M	Parsnips, cooked, boiled, drained, with salt,	246	11%
H	Pasta mix, classic beef, unprepared,	1537	67%
H	Pasta mix, classic cheeseburger macaroni, unprepared,	2152	94%
H	Pasta mix, italian four cheese lasagna, unprepared,	2093	91%
H	Pasta mix, italian lasagna, unprepared,	1850	80%
M	Pasta with sliced franks in tomato sauce, canned entree,	287	12%
M	Pasta with tomato sauce, no meat, canned,	272	12%
M	Pasta, cooked, enriched, with added salt,	131	6%
L	Pasta, cooked, enriched, without added salt,	0	0%
M	Pasta, cooked, unenriched, with added salt,	131	6%
L	Pasta, cooked, unenriched, without added salt,	0	0%
L	Pasta, gluten-free, corn and rice flour, cooked,	0	0%
L	Pasta, gluten-free, corn, cooked,	0	0%
L	Pasta, gluten-free, corn, dry,	0	0%
L	Pasta, homemade, made with egg, cooked,	83	4%
L	Pasta, homemade, made without egg, cooked,	74	3%
L	Pasta, whole grain, 51% whole wheat, remaining enriched semolina, cooked,	0	0%
L	Pasta, whole-wheat, cooked,	0	0%
H	Pastrami, beef, 98% fat-free,	1010	44%

H	Pastrami, turkey,	1123	49%
M	Pastry, pastelitos de guava (guava pastries),	231	10%
H	Pate de foie gras, canned (goose liver pate), smoked,	697	30%
M	Pate, chicken liver, canned,	386	17%
H	Pate, goose liver, smoked, canned,	697	30%
H	Pate, liver, not specified, canned,	697	30%
H	Pate, truffle flavor,	807	35%
L	Peaches, canned, extra light syrup, solids and liquids,	0	0%
L	Peaches, canned, juice pack, solids and liquids,	0	0%
L	Peaches, canned, light syrup pack, solids and liquids,	0	0%
L	Peaches, canned, water pack, solids and liquids,	0	0%
L	Peaches, dehydrated (low-moisture), sulfured, stewed,	0	0%
L	Peaches, dried, sulfured, stewed, with added sugar,	0	0%
L	Peaches, dried, sulfured, stewed, without added sugar,	0	0%
L	Peaches, spiced, canned, heavy syrup pack, solids and liquids,	0	0%
L	Peaches, yellow, raw,	0	0%
M	Peanut butter with omega-3, creamy,	356	15%
H	Peanut butter, chunk style, with salt,	486	21%
M	Peanut butter, chunky, vitamin and mineral fortified,	366	16%
M	Peanut butter, reduced sodium,	203	9%
M	Peanut butter, smooth style, with salt,	426	19%
H	Peanut butter, smooth, reduced fat,	540	23%
M	Peanut butter, smooth, vitamin and mineral fortified,	420	18%
M	Peanut flour, defatted,	180	8%
L	Peanut flour, low fat,	0	0%
M	Peanut spread, reduced sugar,	292	13%
H	Peanuts, all types, cooked, boiled, with salt,	751	33%
M	Peanuts, all types, dry-roasted, with salt,	410	18%
M	Peanuts, all types, oil-roasted, with salt,	320	14%

M	Peanuts, spanish, oil-roasted, with salt,	433	19%
H	Peanuts, valencia, oil-roasted, with salt,	772	34%
L	Peanuts, valencia, raw,	0	0%
M	Peanuts, virginia, oil-roasted, with salt,	433	19%
L	Pear nectar, canned, with added ascorbic acid,	0	0%
L	Pear nectar, canned, without added ascorbic acid,	0	0%
L	Pears, asian, raw,	0	0%
L	Pears, canned, extra heavy syrup pack, solids and liquids,	0	0%
L	Pears, canned, extra light syrup pack, solids and liquids,	0	0%
L	Pears, canned, heavy syrup pack, solids and liquids,	0	0%
L	Pears, canned, heavy syrup, drained,	0	0%
L	Pears, canned, juice pack, solids and liquids,	0	0%
L	Pears, canned, light syrup pack, solids and liquids,	0	0%
L	Pears, canned, water pack, solids and liquids,	0	0%
L	Pears, dried, sulfured, stewed, with added sugar,	0	0%
L	Pears, dried, sulfured, stewed, without added sugar,	0	0%
L	Pears, raw,	0	0%
L	Pears, raw, bartlett,	0	0%
L	Pears, raw, bosc,	0	0%
L	Pears, raw, green anjou,	0	0%
L	Pears, raw, red anjou,	0	0%
L	Peas and carrots, canned, no salt added, solids and liquids,	0	0%
M	Peas and carrots, canned, regular pack, solids and liquids,	260	11%
M	Peas and carrots, frozen, cooked, boiled, drained, with salt,	304	13%
L	Peas and carrots, frozen, cooked, boiled, drained, without salt,	68	3%
L	Peas and carrots, frozen, unprepared,	79	3%
M	Peas and onions, canned, solids and liquids,	442	19%

M	Peas and onions, frozen, cooked, boiled, drained, with salt,	273	12%
L	Peas and onions, frozen, cooked, boiled, drained, without salt,	37	2%
L	Peas and onions, frozen, unprepared,	61	3%
L	Peas, edible-podded, boiled, drained, without salt,	0	0%
M	Peas, edible-podded, cooked, boiled, drained, with salt,	240	10%
M	Peas, edible-podded, frozen, cooked, boiled, drained, with salt,	241	10%
L	Peas, edible-podded, frozen, cooked, boiled, drained, without salt,	0	0%
L	Peas, edible-podded, frozen, unprepared,	0	0%
L	Peas, edible-podded, raw,	0	0%
M	Peas, green (includes baby and lesuer types), canned, drained solids, unprepared,	273	12%
M	Peas, green, canned, drained solids, rinsed in tap water,	231	10%
L	Peas, green, canned, no salt added, drained solids,	0	0%
M	Peas, green, canned, regular pack, solids and liquids,	185	8%
M	Peas, green, canned, seasoned, solids and liquids,	254	11%
M	Peas, green, cooked, boiled, drained, with salt,	239	10%
L	Peas, green, cooked, boiled, drained, without salt,	0	0%
M	Peas, green, frozen, cooked, boiled, drained, with salt,	323	14%
L	Peas, green, frozen, cooked, boiled, drained, without salt,	72	3%
L	Peas, green, frozen, unprepared,	108	5%
L	Peas, green, raw,	0	0%
M	Peas, split, mature seeds, cooked, boiled, with salt,	238	10%
L	Peas, split, mature seeds, cooked, boiled, without salt,	0	0%
M	Pectin, unsweetened, dry mix,	200	9%

L	Pepeao, dried,	70	3%
L	Peppers, ancho, dried,	43	2%
M	Peppers, chili, green, canned,	397	17%
L	Peppers, hot chile, sun-dried,	91	4%
H	Peppers, hot chili, green, canned, pods, excluding seeds, solids and liquids,	1173	51%
H	Peppers, hot chili, red, canned, excluding seeds, solids and liquids,	1173	51%
H	Peppers, hot pickled, canned,	1430	62%
L	Peppers, hungarian, raw,	0	0%
H	Peppers, jalapeno, canned, solids and liquids,	1671	73%
L	Peppers, jalapeno, raw,	0	0%
L	Peppers, pasilla, dried,	89	4%
H	Peppers, sweet, green, canned, solids and liquids,	1369	60%
M	Peppers, sweet, green, cooked, boiled, drained, with salt,	238	10%
L	Peppers, sweet, green, cooked, boiled, drained, without salt,	0	0%
M	Peppers, sweet, green, freeze-dried,	193	8%
M	Peppers, sweet, green, frozen, chopped, cooked, boiled, drained, with salt,	240	10%
L	Peppers, sweet, green, frozen, chopped, unprepared,	0	0%
L	Peppers, sweet, green, raw,	0	0%
H	Peppers, sweet, red, canned, solids and liquids,	1369	60%
M	Peppers, sweet, red, cooked, boiled, drained, with salt,	238	10%
L	Peppers, sweet, red, cooked, boiled, drained, without salt,	0	0%
M	Peppers, sweet, red, freeze-dried,	193	8%
M	Peppers, sweet, red, frozen, chopped, boiled, drained, with salt,	240	10%
L	Peppers, sweet, red, frozen, chopped, boiled, drained, without salt,	0	0%
L	Peppers, sweet, red, frozen, chopped, unprepared,	0	0%
L	Peppers, sweet, red, raw,	0	0%
L	Peppers, sweet, yellow, raw,	0	0%

L	Persimmons, japanese, dried,	0	0%
L	Persimmons, japanese, raw,	0	0%
L	Persimmons, native, raw,	0	0%
L	Pheasant, cooked, total edible,	43	2%
L	Pheasant, leg, meat only, raw,	45	2%
L	Pheasant, raw, meat and skin,	40	2%
L	Pheasant, raw, meat only,	37	2%
H	Phyllo dough,	483	21%
H	Pickle relish, hot dog,	1091	47%
H	Pickle relish, sweet,	811	35%
H	Pickles, chowchow, with cauliflower onion mustard, sweet,	527	23%
H	Pickles, cucumber, dill or kosher dill,	809	35%
H	Pickles, cucumber, sour,	1208	53%
M	Pickles, cucumber, sweet (includes bread and butter pickles),	457	20%
H	Pie crust, cookie-type, chocolate, ready crust,	503	22%
H	Pie crust, cookie-type, prepared from recipe, vanilla wafer, chilled,	515	22%
M	Pie crust, deep dish, frozen, baked, made with enriched flour,	393	17%
M	Pie crust, deep dish, frozen, unbaked, made with enriched flour,	353	15%
H	Pie crust, refrigerated, regular, baked,	472	21%
M	Pie crust, refrigerated, regular, unbaked,	409	18%
H	Pie crust, standard-type, dry mix,	753	33%
H	Pie crust, standard-type, dry mix, prepared, baked,	729	32%
M	Pie crust, standard-type, frozen, ready-to-bake, enriched,	409	18%
M	Pie crust, standard-type, frozen, ready-to-bake, enriched, baked,	467	20%
H	Pie crust, standard-type, frozen, ready-to-bake, unenriched,	576	25%
H	Pie crust, standard-type, prepared from recipe, baked,	542	24%
H	Pie crust, standard-type, prepared from recipe, unbaked,	482	21%
L	Pie fillings, apple, canned,	47	2%

M	Pie, apple, commercially prepared, enriched flour,	201	9%
M	Pie, apple, commercially prepared, unenriched flour,	266	12%
M	Pie, apple, prepared from recipe,	211	9%
M	Pie, banana cream, prepared from mix, no-bake type,	290	13%
M	Pie, banana cream, prepared from recipe,	240	10%
M	Pie, blueberry, commercially prepared,	287	12%
M	Pie, blueberry, prepared from recipe,	185	8%
M	Pie, cherry, commercially prepared,	246	11%
M	Pie, cherry, prepared from recipe,	191	8%
M	Pie, chocolate creme, commercially prepared,	266	12%
M	Pie, chocolate mousse, prepared from mix, no-bake type,	460	20%
M	Pie, coconut cream, prepared from mix, no-bake type,	329	14%
M	Pie, coconut creme, commercially prepared,	204	9%
M	Pie, coconut custard, commercially prepared,	335	15%
M	Pie, dutch apple, commercially prepared,	200	9%
M	Pie, egg custard, commercially prepared,	275	12%
M	Pie, fried pies, cherry,	374	16%
M	Pie, fried pies, fruit,	333	14%
M	Pie, fried pies, lemon,	374	16%
M	Pie, lemon meringue, commercially prepared,	172	7%
M	Pie, lemon meringue, prepared from recipe,	242	11%
M	Pie, mince, prepared from recipe,	254	11%
M	Pie, peach,	217	9%
M	Pie, pecan, commercially prepared,	275	12%
M	Pie, pecan, prepared from recipe,	262	11%
M	Pie, pumpkin, commercially prepared,	239	10%
M	Pie, pumpkin, prepared from recipe,	225	10%
M	Pie, vanilla cream, prepared from recipe,	260	11%
M	Pigeon peas (red gram), mature seeds, cooked, boiled, with salt,	241	10%
L	Pigeon peas (red gram), mature seeds, cooked, boiled, without salt,	0	0%
M	Pigeonpeas, immature seeds, cooked, boiled, drained, with salt,	240	10%

L	Pigeonpeas, immature seeds, cooked, boiled, drained, without salt,	0	0%
L	Pigeonpeas, immature seeds, raw,	0	0%
L	Piki bread, made from blue cornmeal (hopi),	60	3%
L	Pineapple and orange juice drink, canned,	0	0%
L	Pineapple juice, canned or bottled, unsweetened, with added ascorbic acid,	0	0%
L	Pineapple juice, canned or bottled, unsweetened, without added ascorbic acid,	0	0%
L	Pineapple juice, canned, not from concentrate, unsweetened, with added vitamins a, c and e,	0	0%
L	Pineapple juice, frozen concentrate, unsweetened, diluted with 3 volume water,	0	0%
L	Pineapple juice, frozen concentrate, unsweetened, undiluted,	0	0%
L	Pineapple, canned, extra heavy syrup pack, solids and liquids,	0	0%
L	Pineapple, canned, heavy syrup pack, solids and liquids,	0	0%
L	Pineapple, canned, juice pack, drained,	0	0%
L	Pineapple, canned, juice pack, solids and liquids,	0	0%
L	Pineapple, canned, light syrup pack, solids and liquids,	0	0%
L	Pineapple, canned, water pack, solids and liquids,	0	0%
L	Pineapple, frozen, chunks, sweetened,	0	0%
L	Pineapple, raw, all varieties,	0	0%
L	Pineapple, raw, extra sweet variety,	0	0%
L	Pineapple, raw, traditional varieties,	0	0%
L	Pitanga, (surinam-cherry), raw,	0	0%
H	Pizza rolls, frozen, unprepared,	599	26%
M	Pizza, cheese topping, regular crust, frozen, cooked,	447	19%
H	Pizza, cheese topping, rising crust, frozen, cooked,	556	24%
M	Pizza, cheese topping, thin crust, frozen, cooked,	471	20%

H	Pizza, meat and vegetable topping, regular crust, frozen, cooked,	555	24%
H	Pizza, meat and vegetable topping, rising crust, frozen, cooked,	640	28%
H	Pizza, meat topping, thick crust, frozen, cooked,	690	30%
H	Pizza, pepperoni topping, regular crust, frozen, cooked,	590	26%
L	Plantains, cooked,	0	0%
L	Plantains, green, fried,	0	0%
L	Plantains, raw,	0	0%
L	Plums, canned, purple, juice pack, solids and liquids,	0	0%
L	Plums, canned, purple, water pack, solids and liquids,	0	0%
L	Plums, dried (prunes), stewed, with added sugar,	0	0%
L	Plums, dried (prunes), stewed, without added sugar,	0	0%
L	Plums, dried (prunes), uncooked,	0	0%
L	Plums, raw,	0	0%
L	Plums, wild (northern plains indians),	0	0%
M	Pokeberry shoots, (poke), cooked, boiled, drained, with salt,	254	11%
L	Pomegranates, raw,	0	0%
H	Popcorn, microwave, low fat and sodium,	490	21%
H	Popcorn, microwave, regular (butter) flavor, made with palm oil,	763	33%
M	Popcorn, sugar syrup\/caramel, fat-free,	286	12%
H	Popovers, dry mix, enriched,	906	39%
H	Popovers, dry mix, unenriched,	906	39%
L	Potato flour,	55	2%
H	Potato pancakes,	764	33%
M	Potato puffs, frozen, oven-heated,	463	20%
M	Potato puffs, frozen, unprepared,	428	19%
M	Potato salad with egg,	329	14%
H	Potato salad, home-prepared,	529	23%
V.H	Potato soup, instant, dry mix,	2400	104%
M	Potatoes, au gratin, dry mix, prepared with water, whole milk and butter,	439	19%

H	Potatoes, au gratin, dry mix, unprepared,	2095	91%
M	Potatoes, au gratin, home-prepared from recipe using butter,	433	19%
M	Potatoes, au gratin, home-prepared from recipe using margarine,	433	19%
M	Potatoes, baked, flesh, with salt,	241	10%
L	Potatoes, baked, flesh, without salt,	0	0%
M	Potatoes, baked, skin only, with salt,	257	11%
M	Potatoes, boiled, cooked in skin, flesh, with salt,	240	10%
L	Potatoes, boiled, cooked in skin, flesh, without salt,	0	0%
M	Potatoes, boiled, cooked in skin, skin, with salt,	250	11%
M	Potatoes, boiled, cooked without skin, flesh, with salt,	241	10%
L	Potatoes, boiled, cooked without skin, flesh, without salt,	0	0%
M	Potatoes, canned, drained solids,	219	10%
L	Potatoes, canned, drained solids, no salt added,	0	0%
M	Potatoes, canned, solids and liquids,	217	9%
M	Potatoes, french fried, all types, salt added in processing, frozen, home-prepared, oven heated,	324	14%
M	Potatoes, french fried, all types, salt added in processing, frozen, unprepared,	332	14%
L	Potatoes, french fried, cottage-cut, salt not added in processing, frozen, oven-heated,	45	2%
M	Potatoes, french fried, crinkle or regular cut, salt added in processing, frozen, as purchased,	349	15%
M	Potatoes, french fried, crinkle or regular cut, salt added in processing, frozen, oven-heated,	391	17%
M	Potatoes, french fried, cross cut, frozen, unprepared,	393	17%
M	Potatoes, french fried, shoestring, salt added in processing, frozen, as purchased,	323	14%

M	Potatoes, french fried, shoestring, salt added in processing, frozen, oven-heated,	400	17%
M	Potatoes, french fried, steak fries, salt added in processing, frozen, as purchased,	317	14%
M	Potatoes, french fried, steak fries, salt added in processing, frozen, oven-heated,	373	16%
M	Potatoes, french fried, wedge cut, frozen, unprepared,	380	17%
M	Potatoes, frozen, french fried, par fried, cottage-cut, prepared, heated in oven, with salt,	281	12%
H	Potatoes, frozen, french fried, par fried, extruded, prepared, heated in oven, without salt,	613	27%
H	Potatoes, frozen, french fried, par fried, extruded, unprepared,	490	21%
L	Potatoes, hash brown, frozen, with butter sauce, unprepared,	77	3%
M	Potatoes, hash brown, home-prepared,	342	15%
L	Potatoes, hash brown, refrigerated, prepared, pan-fried in canola oil,	77	3%
L	Potatoes, hash brown, refrigerated, unprepared,	42	2%
L	Potatoes, mashed, dehydrated, flakes without milk, dry form,	77	3%
L	Potatoes, mashed, dehydrated, granules with milk, dry form,	82	4%
L	Potatoes, mashed, dehydrated, granules without milk, dry form,	67	3%
M	Potatoes, mashed, dehydrated, prepared from flakes without milk, whole milk and butter added,	164	7%
M	Potatoes, mashed, dehydrated, prepared from flakes without milk, whole milk and margarine added,	332	14%
M	Potatoes, mashed, dehydrated, prepared from granules with milk, water and margarine added,	172	7%

M	Potatoes, mashed, dehydrated, prepared from granules without milk, whole milk and butter added,	257	11%
M	Potatoes, mashed, home-prepared, whole milk added,	302	13%
M	Potatoes, mashed, home-prepared, whole milk and butter added,	317	14%
M	Potatoes, mashed, home-prepared, whole milk and margarine added,	333	14%
M	Potatoes, mashed, prepared from granules, without milk, whole milk and margarine,	263	11%
M	Potatoes, mashed, ready-to-eat,	298	13%
M	Potatoes, microwaved, cooked in skin, flesh, with salt,	243	11%
M	Potatoes, microwaved, cooked, in skin, flesh and skin, with salt,	244	11%
M	Potatoes, microwaved, cooked, in skin, skin with salt,	252	11%
M	Potatoes, o'brien, home-prepared,	217	9%
M	Potatoes, roasted, salt added in processing, frozen, unprepared,	298	13%
L	Potatoes, russet, flesh and skin, raw,	0	0%
M	Potatoes, scalloped, dry mix, prepared with water, whole milk and butter,	341	15%
H	Potatoes, scalloped, dry mix, unprepared,	1578	69%
M	Potatoes, scalloped, home-prepared with butter,	335	15%
M	Potatoes, scalloped, home-prepared with margarine,	335	15%
M	Potatoes, yellow fleshed, french fried, frozen, unprepared,	300	13%
M	Potatoes, yellow fleshed, hash brown, shredded, salt added in processing, frozen, unprepared,	330	14%
M	Potatoes, yellow fleshed, roasted, salt added in processing, frozen, unprepared,	338	15%
H	Poultry salad sandwich spread,	653	28%
L	Poultry, mechanically deboned, from backs and necks with skin, raw,	40	2%

L	Poultry, mechanically deboned, from backs and necks without skin, raw,	51	2%
L	Poultry, mechanically deboned, from mature hens, raw,	40	2%
L	Powerade zero ion4, calorie-free, assorted flavors,	42	2%
L	Prairie turnips, boiled (northern plains indians),	0	0%
L	Prairie turnips, raw (northern plains indians),	0	0%
H	Pretzels, soft,	545	24%
M	Pretzels, soft, unsalted,	252	11%
L	Prickly pears, raw (northern plains indians),	0	0%
L	Prickly pears, raw,	0	0%
H	Protein powder soy based,	733	32%
M	Protein powder whey based,	156	7%
M	Protein supplement, milk based, muscle milk light, powder,	250	11%
M	Protein supplement, milk based, muscle milk, powder,	329	14%
L	Prune juice, canned,	0	0%
L	Prunes, canned, heavy syrup pack, solids and liquids,	0	0%
L	Prunes, dehydrated (low-moisture), stewed,	0	0%
L	Prunes, dehydrated (low-moisture), uncooked,	0	0%
L	Pudding, lemon, dry mix, regular, prepared with sugar, egg yolk and water,	63	3%
V.H	Puddings, all flavors except chocolate, low calorie, instant, dry mix,	3750	163%
H	Puddings, all flavors except chocolate, low calorie, regular, dry mix,	1765	77%
H	Puddings, banana, dry mix, instant,	1499	65%
M	Puddings, banana, dry mix, instant, prepared with 2% milk,	296	13%
M	Puddings, banana, dry mix, instant, prepared with whole milk,	290	13%
H	Puddings, banana, dry mix, instant, with added oil,	1499	65%
H	Puddings, banana, dry mix, regular,	788	34%

M	Puddings, banana, dry mix, regular, prepared with 2% milk,	164	7%
M	Puddings, banana, dry mix, regular, prepared with whole milk,	158	7%
H	Puddings, banana, dry mix, regular, with added oil,	788	34%
V.H	Puddings, chocolate flavor, low calorie, instant, dry mix,	2838	123%
V.H	Puddings, chocolate flavor, low calorie, regular, dry mix,	3326	145%
H	Puddings, chocolate, dry mix, instant,	1771	77%
M	Puddings, chocolate, dry mix, instant, prepared with 2% milk,	284	12%
M	Puddings, chocolate, dry mix, instant, prepared with whole milk,	284	12%
H	Puddings, chocolate, dry mix, regular,	479	21%
L	Puddings, chocolate, dry mix, regular, prepared with 2% milk,	102	4%
L	Puddings, chocolate, dry mix, regular, prepared with whole milk,	98	4%
M	Puddings, chocolate, ready-to-eat,	152	7%
M	Puddings, chocolate, ready-to-eat, fat free,	154	7%
H	Puddings, coconut cream, dry mix, instant,	1040	45%
M	Puddings, coconut cream, dry mix, instant, prepared with 2% milk,	246	11%
M	Puddings, coconut cream, dry mix, instant, prepared with whole milk,	246	11%
H	Puddings, coconut cream, dry mix, regular,	682	30%
M	Puddings, coconut cream, dry mix, regular, prepared with 2% milk,	163	7%
M	Puddings, coconut cream, dry mix, regular, prepared with whole milk,	162	7%
H	Puddings, lemon, dry mix, instant,	1332	58%
M	Puddings, lemon, dry mix, instant, prepared with 2% milk,	268	12%
M	Puddings, lemon, dry mix, instant, prepared with whole milk,	267	12%
H	Puddings, lemon, dry mix, regular,	506	22%
H	Puddings, lemon, dry mix, regular, with added oil, potassium, sodium,	849	37%

M	Puddings, rice, dry mix,	366	16%
L	Puddings, rice, dry mix, prepared with 2% milk,	109	5%
L	Puddings, rice, dry mix, prepared with whole milk,	108	5%
L	Puddings, rice, ready-to-eat,	97	4%
H	Puddings, tapioca, dry mix,	477	21%
L	Puddings, tapioca, dry mix, prepared with 2% milk,	121	5%
L	Puddings, tapioca, dry mix, prepared with whole milk,	120	5%
M	Puddings, tapioca, ready-to-eat,	145	6%
M	Puddings, tapioca, ready-to-eat, fat free,	187	8%
H	Puddings, vanilla, dry mix, instant,	1441	63%
M	Puddings, vanilla, dry mix, instant, prepared with whole milk,	286	12%
H	Puddings, vanilla, dry mix, regular,	635	28%
M	Puddings, vanilla, dry mix, regular, prepared with 2% milk,	159	7%
M	Puddings, vanilla, dry mix, regular, prepared with whole milk,	156	7%
H	Puddings, vanilla, dry mix, regular, with added oil,	754	33%
M	Puddings, vanilla, ready-to-eat,	142	6%
M	Puddings, vanilla, ready-to-eat, fat free,	191	8%
M	Puff pastry, frozen, ready-to-bake,	249	11%
M	Puff pastry, frozen, ready-to-bake, baked,	253	11%
L	Pummelo, raw,	0	0%
L	Pumpkin flowers, raw,	0	0%
M	Pumpkin leaves, cooked, boiled, drained, with salt,	244	11%
M	Pumpkin pie mix, canned,	208	9%
M	Pumpkin, canned, with salt,	241	10%
L	Pumpkin, canned, without salt,	0	0%
M	Pumpkin, cooked, boiled, drained, with salt,	237	10%
L	Pumpkin, cooked, boiled, drained, without salt,	0	0%
M	Pumpkin, flowers, cooked, boiled, drained, with salt,	242	11%
L	Pumpkin, raw,	0	0%

M	Purslane, cooked, boiled, drained, with salt,	280	12%
L	Purslane, cooked, boiled, drained, without salt,	44	2%
L	Purslane, raw,	45	2%
L	Quail, breast, meat only, raw,	55	2%
L	Quail, cooked, total edible,	52	2%
L	Quail, meat and skin, raw,	53	2%
L	Quail, meat only, raw,	51	2%
L	Quinces, raw,	0	0%
L	Quinoa, uncooked,	0	0%
H	Radishes, hawaiian style, pickled,	789	34%
M	Radishes, oriental, cooked, boiled, drained, with salt,	249	11%
M	Radishes, oriental, dried,	278	12%
L	Radishes, raw,	39	2%
L	Raspberries, canned, red, heavy syrup pack, solids and liquids,	0	0%
L	Raspberries, frozen, red, sweetened,	0	0%
L	Raspberries, frozen, unsweetened,	0	0%
L	Raspberries, raw,	0	0%
L	Raspberries, wild (northern plains indians),	0	0%
M	Ravioli, cheese with tomato sauce, frozen, not prepared, includes regular and light entrees,	280	12%
M	Ravioli, cheese-filled, canned,	306	13%
M	Ravioli, meat-filled, with tomato sauce or meat sauce, canned,	283	12%
L	Reddi wip fat free whipped topping,	72	3%
M	Refried beans, canned, fat-free,	438	19%
M	Refried beans, canned, traditional style (includes usda commodity),	370	16%
M	Refried beans, canned, traditional, reduced sodium,	138	6%
M	Refried beans, canned, vegetarian,	430	19%
M	Restaurant, chinese, beef and vegetables,	409	18%
M	Restaurant, chinese, chicken and vegetables,	413	18%
M	Restaurant, chinese, chicken chow mein,	311	14%
M	Restaurant, chinese, egg rolls, assorted,	468	20%
M	Restaurant, chinese, fried rice, without meat,	387	17%

M	Restaurant, chinese, general tso's chicken,	435	19%
M	Restaurant, chinese, kung pao chicken,	402	17%
M	Restaurant, chinese, lemon chicken,	252	11%
H	Restaurant, chinese, orange chicken,	553	24%
H	Restaurant, chinese, sesame chicken,	482	21%
M	Restaurant, chinese, shrimp and vegetables,	375	16%
M	Restaurant, chinese, sweet and sour chicken,	246	11%
M	Restaurant, chinese, vegetable chow mein, without meat or noodles,	344	15%
M	Restaurant, chinese, vegetable lo mein, without meat,	430	19%
H	Restaurant, family style, chicken fingers, from kid's menu,	809	35%
H	Restaurant, family style, chicken tenders,	800	35%
M	Restaurant, family style, chili with meat and beans,	381	17%
M	Restaurant, family style, coleslaw,	221	10%
H	Restaurant, family style, fish fillet, battered or breaded, fried,	561	24%
M	Restaurant, family style, french fries,	357	16%
H	Restaurant, family style, fried mozzarella sticks,	861	37%
M	Restaurant, family style, hash browns,	468	20%
M	Restaurant, family style, macaroni & cheese, from kids' menu,	361	16%
H	Restaurant, family style, onion rings,	692	30%
H	Restaurant, family style, shrimp, breaded and fried,	1125	49%
M	Restaurant, family style, sirloin steak,	339	15%
M	Restaurant, family style, spaghetti and meatballs,	351	15%
M	Restaurant, italian, cheese ravioli with marinara sauce,	306	13%
H	Restaurant, italian, chicken parmesan without pasta,	536	23%
M	Restaurant, italian, lasagna with meat,	466	20%
M	Restaurant, italian, spaghetti with meat sauce,	230	10%
M	Restaurant, italian, spaghetti with pomodoro sauce (no meat),	191	8%

M	Restaurant, latino, arepa (unleavened cornmeal bread),	270	12%
M	Restaurant, latino, arroz con frijoles negros (rice and black beans),	420	18%
H	Restaurant, latino, arroz con grandules (rice and pigeonpeas),	583	25%
M	Restaurant, latino, arroz con habichuelas colorados (rice and red beans),	370	16%
L	Restaurant, latino, arroz con leche (rice pudding),	106	5%
M	Restaurant, latino, black bean soup,	311	14%
M	Restaurant, latino, bunuelos (fried yeast bread),	418	18%
H	Restaurant, latino, chicken and rice, entree, prepared,	518	23%
M	Restaurant, latino, empanadas, beef, prepared,	440	19%
M	Restaurant, latino, pupusas con frijoles (pupusas, bean),	305	13%
M	Restaurant, latino, pupusas con queso (pupusas, cheese),	400	17%
M	Restaurant, latino, tamale, corn,	277	12%
M	Restaurant, latino, tripe soup,	411	18%
H	Restaurant, mexican, cheese enchilada,	528	23%
H	Restaurant, mexican, cheese quesadilla,	701	30%
H	Restaurant, mexican, cheese tamales,	503	22%
M	Restaurant, mexican, refried beans,	376	16%
H	Restaurant, mexican, soft taco with ground beef, cheese and lettuce,	509	22%
H	Restaurant, mexican, spanish rice,	528	23%
L	Rhubarb, frozen, cooked, with sugar,	0	0%
L	Rhubarb, frozen, uncooked,	0	0%
L	Rhubarb, raw,	0	0%
M	Rice and vermicelli mix, beef flavor, prepared with 80% margarine,	364	16%
H	Rice and vermicelli mix, beef flavor, unprepared,	1337	58%
M	Rice and vermicelli mix, chicken flavor, prepared with 80% margarine,	377	16%

H	Rice and vermicelli mix, chicken flavor, unprepared,	1238	54%
M	Rice and vermicelli mix, rice pilaf flavor, prepared with 80% margarine,	430	19%
H	Rice and vermicelli mix, rice pilaf flavor, unprepared,	1303	57%
H	Rice and wheat cereal bar,	500	22%
M	Rice bowl with chicken, frozen entree, prepared (includes fried, teriyaki, and sweet and sour varieties),	333	14%
L	Rice bran, crude,	0	0%
L	Rice cake, cracker (include hain mini rice cakes),	71	3%
L	Rice flour, white, unenriched,	0	0%
L	Rice milk, unsweetened,	39	2%
H	Rice mix, cheese flavor, dry mix, unprepared,	1193	52%
H	Rice mix, white and wild, flavored, unprepared,	1140	50%
M	Rice noodles, dry,	182	8%
L	Rice, brown, long-grain, cooked,	0	0%
L	Rice, brown, long-grain, raw,	0	0%
L	Rice, brown, medium-grain, cooked,	0	0%
L	Rice, brown, medium-grain, raw,	0	0%
L	Rice, white, glutinous, unenriched, cooked,	0	0%
L	Rice, white, long-grain, parboiled, enriched, cooked,	0	0%
L	Rice, white, long-grain, parboiled, enriched, dry,	0	0%
L	Rice, white, long-grain, parboiled, unenriched, cooked,	0	0%
L	Rice, white, long-grain, parboiled, unenriched, dry,	0	0%
L	Rice, white, long-grain, precooked or instant, enriched, prepared,	0	0%
M	Rice, white, long-grain, regular, cooked, enriched, with salt,	382	17%
M	Rice, white, long-grain, regular, cooked, unenriched, with salt,	382	17%
L	Rice, white, long-grain, regular, enriched, cooked,	0	0%

L	Rice, white, long-grain, regular, raw, enriched,	0	0%
L	Rice, white, long-grain, regular, raw, unenriched,	0	0%
L	Rice, white, long-grain, regular, unenriched, cooked without salt,	0	0%
L	Rice, white, medium-grain, cooked, unenriched,	0	0%
L	Rice, white, medium-grain, enriched, cooked,	0	0%
L	Rice, white, medium-grain, raw, enriched,	0	0%
L	Rice, white, medium-grain, raw, unenriched,	0	0%
L	Rice, white, short-grain, cooked, unenriched,	0	0%
L	Rice, white, short-grain, enriched, cooked,	0	0%
L	Rice, white, short-grain, enriched, uncooked,	0	0%
L	Rice, white, short-grain, raw, unenriched,	0	0%
L	Rice, white, steamed, chinese restaurant,	0	0%
H	Rich chocolate, powder,	636	28%
H	Roast beef spread,	724	31%
H	Roast beef, deli style, prepackaged, sliced,	853	37%
H	Rolls, dinner, egg,	566	25%
M	Rolls, dinner, oat bran,	413	18%
M	Rolls, dinner, plain, commercially prepared (includes brown-and-serve),	467	20%
M	Rolls, dinner, plain, prepared from recipe, made with low fat (2%) milk,	415	18%
H	Rolls, dinner, rye,	650	28%
M	Rolls, dinner, sweet,	253	11%
H	Rolls, dinner, wheat,	524	23%
H	Rolls, dinner, whole-wheat,	521	23%
H	Rolls, french,	574	25%
H	Rolls, gluten-free, white, made with brown rice flour, tapioca starch, and potato starch,	707	31%
H	Rolls, gluten-free, white, made with brown rice flour, tapioca starch, and sorghum flour,	544	24%
H	Rolls, gluten-free, white, made with rice flour, rice starch, and corn starch,	593	26%
H	Rolls, gluten-free, whole grain, made with tapioca starch and brown rice flour,	507	22%
H	Rolls, hard (includes kaiser),	544	24%
H	Rolls, pumpernickel,	492	21%

L	Rose hips, wild (northern plains indians),	0	0%
L	Rowal, raw,	0	0%
L	Ruffed grouse, breast meat, skinless, raw,	50	2%
M	Rutabagas, cooked, boiled, drained, with salt,	254	11%
L	Rutabagas, cooked, boiled, drained, without salt,	0	0%
L	Rye flour, dark,	0	0%
L	Rye flour, light,	0	0%
L	Rye flour, medium,	0	0%
L	Rye grain,	0	0%
H	Salad dressing, blue or roquefort cheese dressing, commercial, regular,	642	28%
H	Salad dressing, blue or roquefort cheese dressing, fat-free,	814	35%
H	Salad dressing, blue or roquefort cheese dressing, light,	939	41%
H	Salad dressing, blue or roquefort cheese, low calorie,	939	41%
H	Salad dressing, buttermilk, lite,	1120	49%
H	Salad dressing, caesar dressing, regular,	1209	53%
H	Salad dressing, caesar, fat-free,	1265	55%
H	Salad dressing, caesar, low calorie,	1148	50%
H	Salad dressing, coleslaw dressing, reduced fat,	1600	70%
H	Salad dressing, coleslaw,	710	31%
H	Salad dressing, french dressing, commercial, regular,	836	36%
L	Salad dressing, french dressing, commercial, regular, without salt,	0	0%
H	Salad dressing, french dressing, fat-free,	853	37%
H	Salad dressing, french dressing, reduced calorie,	804	35%
H	Salad dressing, french dressing, reduced fat,	838	36%
H	Salad dressing, french, cottonseed, oil, home recipe,	658	29%
H	Salad dressing, french, home recipe,	658	29%
H	Salad dressing, green goddess, regular,	867	38%
L	Salad dressing, home recipe, vinegar and oil,	0	0%
H	Salad dressing, honey mustard dressing, reduced calorie,	701	30%

H	Salad dressing, honey mustard, regular,	512	22%
H	Salad dressing, italian dressing, commercial, reduced fat,	891	39%
H	Salad dressing, italian dressing, commercial, regular,	993	43%
H	Salad dressing, italian dressing, fat-free,	1129	49%
H	Salad dressing, italian dressing, reduced calorie,	1074	47%
H	Salad dressing, kraft mayo fat free mayonnaise dressing,	750	33%
H	Salad dressing, kraft mayo light mayonnaise,	633	28%
H	Salad dressing, kraft miracle whip free nonfat dressing,	788	34%
H	Salad dressing, mayonnaise and mayonnaise-type, low calorie,	837	36%
H	Salad dressing, mayonnaise type, regular, with salt,	653	28%
H	Salad dressing, mayonnaise-like, fat-free,	788	34%
H	Salad dressing, mayonnaise, imitation, milk cream,	504	22%
M	Salad dressing, mayonnaise, imitation, soybean without cholesterol,	353	15%
H	Salad dressing, mayonnaise, imitation, soybean,	497	22%
H	Salad dressing, mayonnaise, light,	827	36%
H	Salad dressing, mayonnaise, regular,	635	28%
H	Salad dressing, mayonnaise, soybean and safflower oil, with salt,	568	25%
H	Salad dressing, peppercorn dressing, commercial, regular,	1103	48%
H	Salad dressing, poppyseed, creamy,	933	41%
H	Salad dressing, ranch dressing, fat-free,	897	39%
H	Salad dressing, ranch dressing, reduced fat,	1120	49%
H	Salad dressing, ranch dressing, regular,	901	39%
H	Salad dressing, russian dressing,	1133	49%
H	Salad dressing, russian dressing, low calorie,	868	38%
H	Salad dressing, sesame seed dressing, regular,	1000	43%
H	Salad dressing, spray-style dressing, assorted flavors,	1102	48%

M	Salad dressing, sweet and sour,	208	9%
H	Salad dressing, thousand island dressing, fat-free,	788	34%
H	Salad dressing, thousand island dressing, reduced fat,	955	42%
H	Salad dressing, thousand island, commercial, regular,	962	42%
H	Salami, cooked, beef,	1140	50%
H	Salami, cooked, turkey,	1107	48%
H	Salisbury steak with gravy, frozen,	509	22%
L	Salmon, red (sockeye), filets with skin, smoked (alaska native),	51	2%
M	Salmon, sockeye, canned, drained solids, without skin and bones,	386	17%
M	Salmon, sockeye, canned, total can contents,	433	19%
M	Salsify, cooked, boiled, drained, with salt,	252	11%
V.H	Salt, table,	38758	1685%
H	Sandwich spread, meatless,	630	27%
H	Sandwich spread, with chopped pickle, regular, unspecified oils,	1000	43%
H	Sauce, barbecue,	1027	45%
H	Sauce, cheese, ready-to-serve,	828	36%
H	Sauce, cocktail, ready-to-serve,	983	43%
M	Sauce, duck, ready-to-serve,	455	20%
H	Sauce, enchilada, red, mild, ready to serve,	547	24%
V.H	Sauce, fish, ready-to-serve,	7851	341%
H	Sauce, hoisin, ready-to-serve,	1615	70%
M	Sauce, homemade, white, medium,	354	15%
M	Sauce, homemade, white, thick,	373	16%
M	Sauce, homemade, white, thin,	328	14%
H	Sauce, horseradish,	730	32%
H	Sauce, hot chile, sriracha,	2124	92%
V.H	Sauce, oyster, ready-to-serve,	2733	119%
M	Sauce, pasta, spaghetti\/marinara, ready-to-serve,	437	19%
M	Sauce, peanut, made from coconut, water, sugar, peanuts,	319	14%
H	Sauce, peanut, made from peanut butter, water, soy sauce,	1338	58%
H	Sauce, pesto, ready-to-serve, refrigerated,	603	26%

H	Sauce, pesto, ready-to-serve, shelf stable,	998	43%
M	Sauce, pizza, canned, ready-to-serve,	348	15%
H	Sauce, plum, ready-to-serve,	538	23%
V.H	Sauce, ready-to-serve, pepper or hot,	2643	115%
H	Sauce, salsa, ready-to-serve,	711	31%
H	Sauce, salsa, verde, ready-to-serve,	600	26%
H	Sauce, sofrito, prepared from recipe,	1145	50%
H	Sauce, steak, tomato based,	1647	72%
M	Sauce, sweet and sour, ready-to-serve,	371	16%
H	Sauce, tartar, ready-to-serve,	667	29%
V.H	Sauce, teriyaki, ready-to-serve,	3833	167%
H	Sauce, teriyaki, ready-to-serve, reduced sodium,	1778	77%
H	Sauce, tomato chili sauce, bottled, with salt,	1338	58%
H	Sauce, worcestershire,	980	43%
H	Sauerkraut, canned, solids and liquids,	661	29%
H	Sausage, egg and cheese breakfast biscuit,	591	26%
H	Sausage, italian, sweet, links,	570	25%
H	Sausage, italian, turkey, smoked,	928	40%
H	Sausage, meatless,	888	39%
H	Sausage, polish, beef with chicken, hot,	1540	67%
H	Sausage, turkey, breakfast links, mild,	639	28%
H	Sausage, turkey, hot, smoked,	916	40%
H	School lunch, chicken nuggets, whole grain breaded,	511	22%
M	School lunch, chicken patty, whole grain breaded,	467	20%
M	School lunch, pizza, cheese topping, thick crust, whole grain, frozen, cooked,	421	18%
M	School lunch, pizza, cheese topping, thin crust, whole grain, frozen, cooked,	421	18%
H	School lunch, pizza, pepperoni topping, thick crust, whole grain, frozen, cooked,	474	21%
H	School lunch, pizza, pepperoni topping, thin crust, whole grain, frozen, cooked,	495	22%
M	School lunch, pizza, sausage topping, thick crust, whole grain, frozen, cooked,	433	19%
M	School lunch, pizza, sausage topping, thin crust, whole grain, frozen, cooked,	457	20%
V.H	Seasoning mix, dry, chili, original,	4616	201%

V.H	Seasoning mix, dry, sazon, coriander & annatto,	17000	739%
V.H	Seasoning mix, dry, taco, original,	7203	313%
L	Scawccd, irishmoss, raw,	67	3%
M	Seaweed, kelp, raw,	233	10%
L	Seaweed, laver, raw,	48	2%
H	Seaweed, spirulina, dried,	1048	46%
H	Seaweed, wakame, raw,	872	38%
L	Seeds, breadnut tree seeds, dried,	53	2%
L	Seeds, cottonseed meal, partially defatted (glandless),	37	2%
L	Seeds, hemp seed, hulled,	0	0%
L	Seeds, lotus seeds, dried,	0	0%
L	Seeds, lotus seeds, raw,	0	0%
M	Seeds, pumpkin and squash seed kernels, roasted, with salt added,	256	11%
V.H	Seeds, pumpkin and squash seeds, whole, roasted, with salt added,	2541	110%
L	Seeds, safflower seed kernels, dried,	0	0%
L	Seeds, safflower seed meal, partially defatted,	0	0%
L	Seeds, sesame butter, tahini, from raw and stone ground kernels,	74	3%
L	Seeds, sesame butter, tahini, from roasted and toasted kernels (most common type),	115	5%
L	Seeds, sesame butter, tahini, from unroasted kernels (non-chemically removed seed coat),	0	0%
L	Seeds, sesame flour, high-fat,	41	2%
L	Seeds, sesame flour, low-fat,	39	2%
L	Seeds, sesame flour, partially defatted,	41	2%
L	Seeds, sesame meal, partially defatted,	39	2%
L	Seeds, sesame seed kernels, dried (decorticated),	47	2%
H	Seeds, sesame seed kernels, toasted, with salt added (decorticated),	588	26%
L	Seeds, sesame seed kernels, toasted, without salt added (decorticated),	39	2%
L	Seeds, sisymbrium sp. seeds, whole, dried,	92	4%
M	Seeds, sunflower seed butter, with salt added,	331	14%

L	Seeds, sunflower seed butter, without salt,	0	0%
L	Seeds, sunflower seed flour, partially defatted,	0	0%
V.H	Seeds, sunflower seed kernels from shell, dry roasted, with salt added,	6008	261%
H	Seeds, sunflower seed kernels, dry roasted, with salt added,	655	28%
L	Seeds, sunflower seed kernels, dry roasted, without salt,	0	0%
H	Seeds, sunflower seed kernels, oil roasted, with salt added,	733	32%
L	Seeds, sunflower seed kernels, oil roasted, without salt,	0	0%
H	Seeds, sunflower seed kernels, toasted, with salt added,	613	27%
L	Seeds, sunflower seed kernels, toasted, without salt,	0	0%
L	Seeds, watermelon seed kernels, dried,	99	4%
L	Semolina, enriched,	0	0%
L	Semolina, unenriched,	0	0%
M	Sesbania flower, cooked, steamed, with salt,	247	11%
L	Shake, fast food, strawberry,	83	4%
L	Shake, fast food, vanilla,	81	4%
L	Shallots, freeze-dried,	59	3%
L	Sherbet, orange,	46	2%
L	Shortening bread, soybean (hydrogenated) and cottonseed,	0	0%
L	Shortening cake mix, soybean (hydrogenated) and cottonseed (hydrogenated),	0	0%
L	Shortening confectionery, coconut (hydrogenated) and or palm kernel (hydrogenated),	0	0%
L	Shortening frying (heavy duty), beef tallow and cottonseed,	0	0%
L	Shortening frying (heavy duty), palm (hydrogenated),	0	0%
L	Shortening frying (heavy duty), soybean (hydrogenated), linoleic (less than 1%),	0	0%

L	Shortening household soybean (hydrogenated) and palm,	0	0%
L	Shortening industrial, lard and vegetable oil,	0	0%
L	Shortening industrial, soybean (hydrogenated) and cottonseed,	0	0%
L	Shortening, confectionery, fractionated palm,	0	0%
L	Shortening, household, lard and vegetable oil,	0	0%
L	Shortening, household, soybean (partially hydrogenated)-cottonseed (partially hydrogenated),	0	0%
L	Shortening, industrial, soy (partially hydrogenated) and corn for frying,	0	0%
L	Shortening, industrial, soy (partially hydrogenated) for baking and confections,	0	0%
L	Shortening, industrial, soy (partially hydrogenated), pourable liquid fry shortening,	0	0%
L	Shortening, multipurpose, soybean (hydrogenated) and palm (hydrogenated),	0	0%
L	Shortening, special purpose for baking, soybean (hydrogenated) palm and cottonseed,	0	0%
L	Shortening, special purpose for cakes and frostings, soybean (hydrogenated),	0	0%
L	Shortening, vegetable, household, composite,	0	0%
M	Side dishes, potato salad,	328	14%
M	Snack, mixed berry bar,	447	19%
M	Snack, potato chips, made from dried potatoes, plain,	400	17%
H	Snack, pretzel, hard chocolate coated,	494	21%
M	Snacks, bagel chips, plain,	233	10%
V.H	Snacks, beef jerky, chopped and formed,	2081	90%
H	Snacks, beef sticks, smoked,	1531	67%
M	Snacks, brown rice chips,	326	14%
H	Snacks, corn cakes,	488	21%
H	Snacks, corn-based, extruded, chips, barbecue-flavor,	763	33%
H	Snacks, corn-based, extruded, chips, barbecue-flavor, made with enriched masa flour,	763	33%
H	Snacks, corn-based, extruded, chips, plain,	514	22%

H	Snacks, corn-based, extruded, cones, plain,	1022	44%
H	Snacks, corn-based, extruded, onion-flavor,	950	41%
H	Snacks, corn-based, extruded, puffs or twists, cheese-flavor,	942	41%
H	Snacks, corn-based, extruded, puffs or twists, cheese-flavor, unenriched,	896	39%
H	Snacks, cornnuts, barbecue-flavor,	600	26%
M	Snacks, crisped rice bar, almond,	234	10%
M	Snacks, crisped rice bar, chocolate chip,	278	12%
M	Snacks, fruit leather, pieces,	403	18%
M	Snacks, fruit leather, pieces, with vitamin c,	317	14%
M	Snacks, fruit leather, rolls,	317	14%
M	Snacks, granola bar, with coconut, chocolate coated,	152	7%
M	Snacks, granola bars, hard, almond,	256	11%
M	Snacks, granola bars, hard, chocolate chip,	344	15%
M	Snacks, granola bars, hard, peanut butter,	283	12%
M	Snacks, granola bars, hard, plain,	294	13%
H	Snacks, granola bars, soft, almond, confectioners coating,	486	21%
M	Snacks, granola bars, soft, coated, milk chocolate coating, chocolate chip,	200	9%
M	Snacks, granola bars, soft, coated, milk chocolate coating, peanut butter,	193	8%
M	Snacks, granola bars, soft, uncoated, chocolate chip,	251	11%
M	Snacks, granola bars, soft, uncoated, nut and raisin,	254	11%
M	Snacks, granola bars, soft, uncoated, peanut butter and chocolate chip,	328	14%
M	Snacks, granola bars, soft, uncoated, peanut butter,	409	18%
M	Snacks, granola bars, soft, uncoated, plain,	278	12%
M	Snacks, granola bars, soft, uncoated, raisin,	282	12%
M	Snacks, granola bites, mixed flavors,	167	7%
M	Snacks, oriental mix, rice-based,	413	18%
H	Snacks, pita chips, salted,	854	37%
M	Snacks, plantain chips, salted,	202	9%
L	Snacks, popcorn, air-popped (unsalted),	0	0%
M	Snacks, popcorn, cakes,	288	13%

M	Snacks, popcorn, caramel-coated, with peanuts,	177	8%
M	Snacks, popcorn, caramel-coated, without peanuts,	206	9%
H	Snacks, popcorn, cheese-flavor,	889	39%
L	Snacks, popcorn, home-prepared, oil-popped, unsalted,	0	0%
H	Snacks, popcorn, microwave, 94% fat free,	571	25%
H	Snacks, popcorn, microwave, low fat,	540	23%
H	Snacks, popcorn, microwave, regular (butter) flavor, made with partially hydrogenated oil,	764	33%
H	Snacks, popcorn, oil-popped, microwave, regular flavor, no trans fat,	679	30%
H	Snacks, popcorn, oil-popped, white popcorn, salt added,	884	38%
H	Snacks, potato chips, barbecue-flavor,	545	24%
M	Snacks, potato chips, cheese-flavor,	458	20%
H	Snacks, potato chips, fat free, salted,	643	28%
H	Snacks, potato chips, fat-free, made with olestra,	554	24%
M	Snacks, potato chips, lightly salted,	187	8%
H	Snacks, potato chips, made from dried potatoes (preformed), multigrain,	544	24%
H	Snacks, potato chips, made from dried potatoes, cheese-flavor,	600	26%
M	Snacks, potato chips, made from dried potatoes, fat-free, made with olestra,	429	19%
M	Snacks, potato chips, made from dried potatoes, reduced fat,	450	20%
H	Snacks, potato chips, made from dried potatoes, sour-cream and onion-flavor,	541	24%
H	Snacks, potato chips, plain, made with partially hydrogenated soybean oil, salted,	594	26%
H	Snacks, potato chips, plain, salted,	527	23%
H	Snacks, potato chips, reduced fat,	492	21%
H	Snacks, potato chips, sour-cream-and-onion-flavor,	549	24%
H	Snacks, potato chips, white, restructured, baked,	554	24%
H	Snacks, potato sticks,	633	28%

H	Snacks, pretzels, hard, confectioner's coating, chocolate-flavor,	569	25%
M	Snacks, pretzels, hard, plain, made with enriched flour, unsalted,	250	11%
H	Snacks, pretzels, hard, plain, made with unenriched flour, salted,	1715	75%
M	Snacks, pretzels, hard, plain, made with unenriched flour, unsalted,	289	13%
H	Snacks, pretzels, hard, plain, salted,	1240	54%
M	Snacks, pretzels, hard, whole-wheat including both salted and unsalted,	203	9%
L	Snacks, rice cakes, brown rice, buckwheat,	116	5%
L	Snacks, rice cakes, brown rice, buckwheat, unsalted,	0	0%
M	Snacks, rice cakes, brown rice, corn,	167	7%
M	Snacks, rice cakes, brown rice, multigrain,	252	11%
L	Snacks, rice cakes, brown rice, multigrain, unsalted,	0	0%
L	Snacks, rice cakes, brown rice, rye,	110	5%
M	Snacks, rice cakes, brown rice, sesame seed,	227	10%
L	Snacks, rice cakes, brown rice, sesame seed, unsalted,	0	0%
M	Snacks, rice cracker brown rice, plain,	326	14%
H	Snacks, sesame sticks, wheat-based, salted,	1488	65%
H	Snacks, soy chips or crisps, salted,	842	37%
M	Snacks, taro chips,	342	15%
H	Snacks, tortilla chips, light (baked with less oil),	564	25%
H	Snacks, tortilla chips, low fat, made with olestra, nacho cheese,	705	31%
H	Snacks, tortilla chips, nacho cheese,	691	30%
H	Snacks, tortilla chips, nacho-flavor, made with enriched masa flour,	708	31%
H	Snacks, tortilla chips, nacho-flavor, reduced fat,	1003	44%
M	Snacks, tortilla chips, plain, white corn, salted,	328	14%
H	Snacks, tortilla chips, ranch-flavor,	519	23%
H	Snacks, tortilla chips, taco-flavor,	787	34%
M	Snacks, trail mix, regular,	229	10%

L	Snacks, trail mix, regular, with chocolate chips, salted nuts and seeds,	121	5%
L	Snacks, trail mix, tropical,	95	4%
M	Snacks, vegetable chips, made from garden vegetables,	357	16%
M	Snacks, yucca (cassava) chips, salted,	296	13%
L	Sorghum flour, refined, unenriched,	0	0%
L	Sorghum flour, whole-grain,	0	0%
L	Sorghum grain,	0	0%
H	Soup, bean with frankfurters, canned, condensed,	831	36%
M	Soup, bean with frankfurters, canned, prepared with equal volume water,	437	19%
M	Soup, beef and vegetables, canned, ready-to-serve,	326	14%
M	Soup, beef and vegetables, reduced sodium, canned, ready-to-serve,	175	8%
M	Soup, beef barley, ready to serve,	297	13%
H	Soup, beef broth bouillon and consomme, canned, condensed,	694	30%
M	Soup, beef broth or bouillon canned, ready-to-serve,	372	16%
V.H	Soup, beef broth or bouillon, powder, dry,	26000	1130%
M	Soup, beef broth or bouillon, powder, prepared with water,	382	17%
M	Soup, beef broth, bouillon, consomme, prepared with equal volume water,	264	11%
V.H	Soup, beef broth, cubed, dry,	24000	1043%
M	Soup, beef broth, cubed, prepared with water,	260	11%
M	Soup, beef broth, less\reduced sodium, ready to serve,	225	10%
H	Soup, beef mushroom, canned, condensed,	709	31%
M	Soup, beef mushroom, canned, prepared with equal volume water,	386	17%
H	Soup, beef noodle, canned, condensed,	653	28%
M	Soup, beef noodle, canned, prepared with equal volume water,	325	14%
M	Soup, beef stroganoff, canned, chunky style, ready-to-serve,	435	19%

H	Soup, beef with vegetables and barley, canned, condensed, single brand,	707	31%
H	Soup, black bean, canned, condensed,	970	42%
H	Soup, black bean, canned, prepared with equal volume water,	487	21%
H	Soup, bouillon cubes and granules, low sodium, dry,	1067	46%
H	Soup, broccoli cheese, canned, condensed, commercial,	661	29%
H	Soup, cheese, canned, condensed,	692	30%
M	Soup, cheese, canned, prepared with equal volume milk,	406	18%
M	Soup, cheese, canned, prepared with equal volume water,	388	17%
M	Soup, chicken and vegetable, canned, ready-to-serve,	229	10%
V.H	Soup, chicken broth cubes, dry,	24000	1043%
M	Soup, chicken broth cubes, dry, prepared with water,	326	14%
V.H	Soup, chicken broth or bouillon, dry,	23875	1038%
M	Soup, chicken broth or bouillon, dry, prepared with water,	401	17%
H	Soup, chicken broth, canned, condensed,	621	27%
M	Soup, chicken broth, canned, prepared with equal volume water,	306	13%
M	Soup, chicken broth, less\/reduced sodium, ready to serve,	231	10%
M	Soup, chicken broth, ready-to-serve,	371	16%
M	Soup, chicken corn chowder, chunky, ready-to-serve, single brand,	299	13%
H	Soup, chicken gumbo, canned, condensed,	693	30%
M	Soup, chicken gumbo, canned, prepared with equal volume water,	391	17%
M	Soup, chicken mushroom chowder, chunky, ready-to-serve, single brand,	339	15%
H	Soup, chicken mushroom, canned, condensed,	669	29%
M	Soup, chicken mushroom, canned, prepared with equal volume water,	327	14%
H	Soup, chicken noodle, canned, condensed,	681	30%

M	Soup, chicken noodle, canned, prepared with equal volume water,	335	15%
V,H	Soup, chicken noodle, dry, mix,	3643	158%
M	Soup, chicken noodle, dry, mix, prepared with water,	229	10%
M	Soup, chicken noodle, low sodium, canned, prepared with equal volume water,	173	8%
M	Soup, chicken noodle, reduced sodium, canned, ready-to-serve,	186	8%
M	Soup, chicken rice, canned, chunky, ready-to-serve,	370	16%
M	Soup, chicken vegetable with potato and cheese, chunky, ready-to-serve,	416	18%
H	Soup, chicken vegetable, canned, condensed,	706	31%
M	Soup, chicken vegetable, chunky, reduced fat, reduced sodium, ready-to-serve, single brand,	192	8%
H	Soup, chicken with rice, canned, condensed,	645	28%
M	Soup, chicken with rice, canned, prepared with equal volume water,	238	10%
H	Soup, chicken with star-shaped pasta, canned, condensed, single brand,	732	32%
M	Soup, chicken, canned, chunky, ready-to-serve,	354	15%
H	Soup, chili beef, canned, condensed,	788	34%
M	Soup, chili beef, canned, prepared with equal volume water,	388	17%
M	Soup, chunky beef, canned, ready-to-serve,	338	15%
M	Soup, chunky chicken noodle, canned, ready-to-serve,	306	13%
M	Soup, chunky vegetable, canned, ready-to-serve,	267	12%
M	Soup, chunky vegetable, reduced sodium, canned, ready-to-serve,	138	6%
M	Soup, clam chowder, manhattan style, canned, chunky, ready-to-serve,	417	18%
H	Soup, clam chowder, manhattan, canned, condensed,	698	30%

M	Soup, clam chowder, manhattan, canned, prepared with equal volume water,	226	10%
H	Soup, clam chowder, new england, canned, condensed,	516	22%
M	Soup, clam chowder, new england, canned, prepared with equal volume low fat (2%) milk,	273	12%
M	Soup, clam chowder, new england, canned, prepared with equal volume water,	254	11%
M	Soup, clam chowder, new england, canned, ready-to-serve,	343	15%
M	Soup, clam chowder, new england, reduced sodium, canned, ready-to-serve,	194	8%
H	Soup, cream of asparagus, canned, condensed,	669	29%
M	Soup, cream of asparagus, canned, prepared with equal volume milk,	420	18%
M	Soup, cream of asparagus, canned, prepared with equal volume water,	402	17%
H	Soup, cream of celery, canned, condensed,	516	22%
M	Soup, cream of celery, canned, prepared with equal volume milk,	272	12%
M	Soup, cream of celery, canned, prepared with equal volume water,	254	11%
H	Soup, cream of chicken, canned, condensed,	702	31%
M	Soup, cream of chicken, canned, condensed, reduced sodium,	357	16%
H	Soup, cream of chicken, canned, condensed, single brand,	788	34%
M	Soup, cream of chicken, canned, prepared with equal volume milk,	362	16%
M	Soup, cream of chicken, canned, prepared with equal volume water,	347	15%
M	Soup, cream of chicken, dry, mix, prepared with water,	454	20%
H	Soup, cream of mushroom, canned, condensed,	691	30%
M	Soup, cream of mushroom, canned, condensed, reduced sodium,	383	17%
M	Soup, cream of mushroom, canned, prepared with equal volume low fat (2%) milk,	357	16%

M	Soup, cream of mushroom, canned, prepared with equal volume water,	340	15%
H	Soup, cream of onion, canned, condensed,	637	28%
M	Soup, cream of onion, canned, prepared with equal volume milk,	405	18%
M	Soup, cream of onion, canned, prepared with equal volume water,	380	17%
H	Soup, cream of potato, canned, condensed,	604	26%
M	Soup, cream of potato, canned, prepared with equal volume milk,	230	10%
M	Soup, cream of potato, canned, prepared with equal volume water,	238	10%
H	Soup, cream of shrimp, canned, condensed,	685	30%
M	Soup, cream of shrimp, canned, prepared with equal volume low fat (2%) milk,	354	15%
M	Soup, cream of shrimp, canned, prepared with equal volume water,	391	17%
V.H	Soup, cream of vegetable, dry, powder,	4957	216%
M	Soup, egg drop, chinese restaurant,	370	16%
M	Soup, hot and sour, chinese restaurant,	376	16%
M	Soup, minestrone, canned, chunky, ready-to-serve,	288	13%
H	Soup, minestrone, canned, condensed,	516	22%
M	Soup, minestrone, canned, prepared with equal volume water,	254	11%
M	Soup, minestrone, canned, reduced sodium, ready-to-serve,	215	9%
H	Soup, mushroom barley, canned, condensed,	573	25%
M	Soup, mushroom barley, canned, prepared with equal volume water,	365	16%
H	Soup, mushroom with beef stock, canned, condensed,	773	34%
M	Soup, mushroom with beef stock, canned, prepared with equal volume water,	397	17%
H	Soup, onion, canned, condensed,	516	22%
V.H	Soup, onion, dry, mix,	8031	349%
M	Soup, onion, dry, mix, prepared with water,	346	15%
H	Soup, oyster stew, canned, condensed,	722	31%
M	Soup, oyster stew, canned, prepared with equal volume milk,	425	18%

M	Soup, oyster stew, canned, prepared with equal volume water,	407	18%
H	Soup, pea, green, canned, condensed,	680	30%
M	Soup, pea, green, canned, prepared with equal volume milk,	352	15%
M	Soup, pea, green, canned, prepared with equal volume water,	336	15%
M	Soup, progresso, beef barley, traditional, ready to serve,	284	12%
H	Soup, ramen noodle, any flavor, dry,	1855	81%
H	Soup, ramen noodle, beef flavor, dry,	1727	75%
H	Soup, ramen noodle, chicken flavor, dry,	1923	84%
H	Soup, ramen noodle, dry, any flavor, reduced fat, reduced sodium,	1200	52%
H	Soup, shark fin, restaurant-prepared,	501	22%
M	Soup, sirloin burger with vegetables, ready-to-serve, single brand,	361	16%
M	Soup, stock, beef, home-prepared,	198	9%
M	Soup, stock, chicken, home-prepared,	143	6%
M	Soup, stock, fish, home-prepared,	156	7%
H	Soup, tomato beef with noodle, canned, condensed,	731	32%
M	Soup, tomato beef with noodle, canned, prepared with equal volume water,	367	16%
H	Soup, tomato bisque, canned, condensed,	698	30%
M	Soup, tomato bisque, canned, prepared with equal volume milk,	442	19%
M	Soup, tomato bisque, canned, prepared with equal volume water,	424	18%
H	Soup, tomato rice, canned, condensed,	635	28%
M	Soup, tomato rice, canned, prepared with equal volume water,	319	14%
M	Soup, tomato, canned, condensed,	377	16%
M	Soup, tomato, canned, prepared with equal volume low fat (2%) milk,	206	9%
M	Soup, tomato, canned, prepared with equal volume water, commercial,	186	8%
M	Soup, tomato, dry, mix, prepared with water,	356	15%
M	Soup, turkey noodle, canned, prepared with equal volume water,	334	15%

M	Soup, turkey vegetable, canned, prepared with equal volume water,	376	16%
M	Soup, turkey, chunky, canned, ready-to-serve,	391	17%
H	Soup, vegetable beef, canned, condensed,	706	31%
H	Soup, vegetable beef, canned, condensed, single brand,	555	24%
M	Soup, vegetable beef, canned, prepared with equal volume water,	349	15%
M	Soup, vegetable beef, microwavable, ready-to-serve, single brand,	376	16%
M	Soup, vegetable broth, ready to serve,	296	13%
M	Soup, vegetable soup, condensed, low sodium, prepared with equal volume water,	194	8%
H	Soup, vegetable with beef broth, canned, condensed,	515	22%
M	Soup, vegetable with beef broth, canned, prepared with equal volume water,	253	11%
M	Soup, vegetable, canned, low sodium, condensed,	385	17%
H	Soup, vegetarian vegetable, canned, condensed,	516	22%
M	Soup, vegetarian vegetable, canned, prepared with equal volume water,	338	15%
M	Soup, wonton, chinese restaurant,	406	18%
M	Sour cream, fat free,	141	6%
L	Sour cream, imitation, cultured,	102	4%
L	Sour cream, light,	83	4%
L	Sour cream, reduced fat,	70	3%
L	Sour dressing, non-butterfat, cultured, filled cream-type,	48	2%
L	Soy meal, defatted, raw,	0	0%
H	Soy protein concentrate, produced by acid wash,	900	39%
L	Soy protein concentrate, produced by alcohol extraction,	0	0%
H	Soy protein isolate,	1005	44%
L	Soy protein isolate, potassium type,	50	2%
V.H	Soy sauce made from hydrolyzed vegetable protein,	6820	297%

V.H	Soy sauce made from soy (tamari),	5586	243%
V.H	Soy sauce made from soy and wheat (shoyu),	5493	239%
V.H	Soy sauce made from soy and wheat (shoyu), low sodium,	3598	156%
V.H	Soy sauce, reduced sodium, made from hydrolyzed vegetable protein,	2890	126%
M	Soybeans, green, cooked, boiled, drained, with salt,	250	11%
L	Soybeans, mature cooked, boiled, without salt,	0	0%
M	Soybeans, mature seeds, cooked, boiled, with salt,	237	10%
L	Soybeans, mature seeds, dry roasted,	0	0%
L	Soybeans, mature seeds, raw,	0	0%
L	Soybeans, mature seeds, roasted, no salt added,	0	0%
M	Soybeans, mature seeds, roasted, salted,	163	7%
M	Soybeans, mature seeds, sprouted, cooked, steamed, with salt,	246	11%
L	Soymilk (all flavors), enhanced,	50	2%
L	Soymilk (all flavors), lowfat, with added calcium, vitamins a and d,	37	2%
L	Soymilk (all flavors), nonfat, with added calcium, vitamins a and d,	57	2%
L	Soymilk (all flavors), unsweetened, with added calcium, vitamins a and d,	37	2%
L	Soymilk, chocolate and other flavors, light, with added calcium, vitamins a and d,	46	2%
L	Soymilk, chocolate, nonfat, with added calcium, vitamins a and d,	57	2%
L	Soymilk, chocolate, unfortified,	53	2%
L	Soymilk, chocolate, with added calcium, vitamins a and d,	53	2%
L	Soymilk, original and vanilla, light, unsweetened, with added calcium, vitamins a and d,	63	3%
L	Soymilk, original and vanilla, light, with added calcium, vitamins a and d,	48	2%
L	Soymilk, original and vanilla, unfortified,	51	2%

L	Soymilk, original and vanilla, with added calcium, vitamins a and d,	47	2%
M	Spaghetti with meat sauce, frozen entree,	238	10%
L	Spaghetti, protein-fortified, cooked, enriched (n x 6.25),	0	0%
L	Spaghetti, spinach, dry,	36	2%
M	Spaghetti, with meatballs in tomato sauce, canned,	280	12%
M	Spanish rice mix, dry mix, prepared (with canola\/vegetable oil blend or diced tomatoes and margarine),	349	15%
H	Spanish rice mix, dry mix, unprepared,	1085	47%
M	Spearmint, dried,	344	15%
L	Spelt, cooked,	0	0%
L	Spices, allspice, ground,	77	3%
L	Spices, basil, dried,	76	3%
M	Spices, celery seed,	160	7%
L	Spices, chervil, dried,	83	4%
V.H	Spices, chili powder,	2867	125%
M	Spices, cloves, ground,	277	12%
M	Spices, coriander leaf, dried,	211	9%
M	Spices, cumin seed,	168	7%
L	Spices, curry powder,	52	2%
M	Spices, dill weed, dried,	208	9%
L	Spices, fennel seed,	88	4%
L	Spices, fenugreek seed,	67	3%
L	Spices, garlic powder,	60	3%
L	Spices, mace, ground,	80	3%
L	Spices, marjoram, dried,	77	3%
L	Spices, onion powder,	73	3%
L	Spices, paprika,	68	3%
M	Spices, parsley, dried,	452	20%
L	Spices, pepper, white,	0	0%
L	Spices, pumpkin pie spice,	52	2%
L	Spices, rosemary, dried,	50	2%
M	Spices, saffron,	148	6%
L	Spices, tarragon, dried,	62	3%
L	Spices, thyme, dried,	55	2%
H	Spinach souffle,	566	25%

L	Spinach, canned, no salt added, solids and liquids,	75	3%
M	Spinach, canned, regular pack, drained solids,	322	14%
M	Spinach, canned, regular pack, solids and liquids,	319	14%
M	Spinach, cooked, boiled, drained, with salt,	306	13%
L	Spinach, cooked, boiled, drained, without salt,	70	3%
M	Spinach, frozen, chopped or leaf, cooked, boiled, drained, with salt,	322	14%
L	Spinach, frozen, chopped or leaf, cooked, boiled, drained, without salt,	97	4%
L	Spinach, frozen, chopped or leaf, unprepared,	74	3%
L	Spinach, raw,	79	3%
M	Split pea soup, canned, reduced sodium, prepared with water or ready-to serve,	166	7%
L	Squab, (pigeon), light meat without skin, raw,	55	2%
L	Squab, (pigeon), meat and skin, raw,	54	2%
L	Squab, (pigeon), meat only, raw,	51	2%
M	Squash, summer, all varieties, cooked, boiled, drained, with salt,	237	10%
L	Squash, summer, all varieties, cooked, boiled, drained, without salt,	0	0%
L	Squash, summer, all varieties, raw,	0	0%
L	Squash, summer, crookneck and straightneck, canned, drained, solid, without salt,	0	0%
M	Squash, summer, crookneck and straightneck, cooked, boiled, drained, with salt,	237	10%
L	Squash, summer, crookneck and straightneck, cooked, boiled, drained, without salt,	0	0%
M	Squash, summer, crookneck and straightneck, frozen, cooked, boiled, drained, with salt,	242	11%
L	Squash, summer, crookneck and straightneck, frozen, unprepared,	0	0%
L	Squash, summer, crookneck and straightneck, raw,	0	0%

M	Squash, summer, scallop, cooked, boiled, drained, with salt,	237	10%
L	Squash, summer, scallop, cooked, boiled, drained, without salt,	0	0%
L	Squash, summer, scallop, raw,	0	0%
M	Squash, winter, acorn, cooked, baked, with salt,	240	10%
L	Squash, winter, acorn, cooked, baked, without salt,	0	0%
M	Squash, winter, acorn, cooked, boiled, mashed, with salt,	239	10%
L	Squash, winter, acorn, cooked, boiled, mashed, without salt,	0	0%
L	Squash, winter, acorn, raw,	0	0%
M	Squash, winter, all varieties, cooked, baked, with salt,	237	10%
L	Squash, winter, all varieties, cooked, baked, without salt,	0	0%
L	Squash, winter, all varieties, raw,	0	0%
M	Squash, winter, butternut, cooked, baked, with salt,	240	10%
L	Squash, winter, butternut, cooked, baked, without salt,	0	0%
M	Squash, winter, butternut, frozen, cooked, boiled, with salt,	238	10%
L	Squash, winter, butternut, frozen, cooked, boiled, without salt,	0	0%
L	Squash, winter, butternut, frozen, unprepared,	0	0%
L	Squash, winter, butternut, raw,	0	0%
M	Squash, winter, hubbard, baked, with salt,	244	11%
M	Squash, winter, hubbard, cooked, boiled, mashed, with salt,	241	10%
L	Squash, winter, hubbard, cooked, boiled, mashed, without salt,	0	0%
M	Squash, winter, spaghetti, cooked, boiled, drained, or baked, with salt,	254	11%
L	Stew, dumpling with mutton (navajo),	46	2%
L	Stew, hominy with mutton (navajo),	45	2%
L	Stew, mutton, corn, squash (navajo),	49	2%

L	Stew, pinto bean and hominy, badufsuki (hopi),	45	2%
L	Stinging nettles, blanched (northern plains indians),	0	0%
L	Strawberries, canned, heavy syrup pack, solids and liquids,	0	0%
L	Strawberries, frozen, sweetened, sliced,	0	0%
L	Strawberries, frozen, sweetened, whole,	0	0%
L	Strawberries, frozen, unsweetened,	0	0%
L	Strawberries, raw,	0	0%
L	Strawberry-flavor beverage mix, powder,	38	2%
L	Strawberry-flavor beverage mix, powder, prepared with whole milk,	48	2%
M	Strudel, apple,	135	6%
M	Succotash, (corn and limas), canned, with cream style corn,	245	11%
M	Succotash, (corn and limas), canned, with whole kernel corn, solids and liquids,	221	10%
M	Succotash, (corn and limas), cooked, boiled, drained, with salt,	253	11%
M	Succotash, (corn and limas), frozen, cooked, boiled, drained, with salt,	281	12%
L	Succotash, (corn and limas), frozen, cooked, boiled, drained, without salt,	45	2%
L	Succotash, (corn and limas), frozen, unprepared,	45	2%
L	Sugar, turbinado,	0	0%
L	Sugars, granulated,	0	0%
L	Sugars, powdered,	0	0%
M	Swamp cabbage (skunk cabbage), cooked, boiled, drained, with salt,	358	16%
L	Swamp cabbage (skunk cabbage), cooked, boiled, drained, without salt,	122	5%
L	Swamp cabbage, (skunk cabbage), raw,	113	5%
M	Sweet potato leaves, cooked, steamed, with salt,	249	11%
M	Sweet potato puffs, frozen, unprepared,	250	11%
L	Sweet potato, canned, mashed,	75	3%
L	Sweet potato, canned, syrup pack, drained solids,	39	2%

L	Sweet potato, canned, vacuum pack,	53	2%
M	Sweet potato, cooked, baked in skin, flesh, with salt,	246	11%
L	Sweet potato, cooked, baked in skin, flesh, without salt,	36	2%
M	Sweet potato, cooked, boiled, without skin, with salt,	263	11%
L	Sweet potato, cooked, candied, home-prepared,	119	5%
M	Sweet potato, frozen, cooked, baked, with salt,	244	11%
L	Sweet potato, raw, unprepared,	55	2%
M	Sweet potatoes, french fried, crosscut, frozen, unprepared,	214	9%
M	Sweet potatoes, french fried, frozen as packaged, salt added in processing,	146	6%
M	Sweet rolls, cheese,	357	16%
M	Sweet rolls, cinnamon, commercially prepared with raisins,	304	13%
H	Sweet rolls, cinnamon, refrigerated dough with frosting,	765	33%
H	Sweet rolls, cinnamon, refrigerated dough with frosting, baked,	832	36%
L	Sweetener, herbal extract powder from stevia leaf,	0	0%
L	Sweetener, syrup, agave,	0	0%
L	Sweeteners, for baking, contains sugar and sucralose,	0	0%
H	Sweeteners, sugar substitute, granulated, brown,	572	25%
L	Sweeteners, tabletop, fructose, liquid,	0	0%
M	Sweeteners, tabletop, saccharin (sodium saccharin),	428	19%
L	Syrup, cane,	58	3%
L	Syrup, fruit flavored,	0	0%
L	Syrups, chocolate, hershey's genuine chocolate flavored lite syrup,	100	4%
M	Syrups, corn, dark,	155	7%
L	Syrups, corn, high-fructose,	0	0%
L	Syrups, corn, light,	62	3%

M	Syrups, sugar free,	210	9%
L	Syrups, table blends, cane and 15% maple,	104	5%
L	Syrups, table blends, corn, refiner, and sugar,	71	3%
L	Syrups, table blends, pancake,	82	4%
M	Syrups, table blends, pancake, reduced-calorie,	178	8%
L	Syrups, table blends, pancake, with 2% maple,	61	3%
L	Syrups, table blends, pancake, with 2% maple, with added potassium,	61	3%
M	Syrups, table blends, pancake, with butter,	287	12%
M	Taco shells, baked,	324	14%
M	Tamales (navajo),	427	19%
L	Tangerine juice, canned, sweetened,	0	0%
L	Tangerine juice, raw,	0	0%
L	Tangerines, (mandarin oranges), canned, juice pack,	0	0%
L	Tangerines, (mandarin oranges), canned, juice pack, drained,	0	0%
L	Tangerines, (mandarin oranges), raw,	0	0%
L	Tapioca, pearl, dry,	0	0%
M	Taquitos, frozen, beef and cheese, oven-heated,	456	20%
M	Taquitos, frozen, chicken and cheese, oven-heated,	453	20%
L	Taro leaves, cooked, steamed, without salt,	0	0%
L	Taro leaves, raw,	0	0%
L	Taro shoots, cooked, without salt,	0	0%
L	Taro shoots, raw,	0	0%
M	Taro, cooked, with salt,	251	11%
M	Taro, leaves, cooked, steamed, with salt,	238	10%
M	Taro, shoots, cooked, with salt,	238	10%
M	Taro, tahitian, cooked, with salt,	290	13%
L	Taro, tahitian, cooked, without salt,	54	2%
L	Taro, tahitian, raw,	50	2%
L	Tea, black, brewed, prepared with distilled water,	0	0%
L	Tea, black, brewed, prepared with tap water,	0	0%
L	Tea, black, brewed, prepared with tap water, decaffeinated,	0	0%

L	Tea, black, ready to drink,	0	0%
L	Tea, black, ready to drink, decaffeinated, diet,	0	0%
L	Tea, black, ready-to-drink, lemon, sweetened,	0	0%
L	Tea, black, ready-to-drink, peach, diet,	0	0%
L	Tea, green, brewed, decaffeinated,	0	0%
L	Tea, green, brewed, regular,	0	0%
L	Tea, green, instant, decaffeinated, lemon, unsweetened, fortified with vitamin c,	0	0%
L	Tea, green, ready to drink, ginseng and honey, sweetened,	0	0%
L	Tea, hibiscus, brewed,	0	0%
M	Tea, instant, decaffeinated, lemon, diet,	412	18%
L	Tea, instant, decaffeinated, lemon, sweetened,	0	0%
L	Tea, instant, decaffeinated, unsweetened,	72	3%
L	Tea, instant, lemon, sweetened, powder,	0	0%
L	Tea, instant, lemon, sweetened, prepared with water,	0	0%
L	Tea, instant, lemon, unsweetened,	55	2%
L	Tea, instant, lemon, with added ascorbic acid,	0	0%
M	Tea, instant, sweetened with sodium saccharin, lemon-flavored, powder,	412	18%
L	Tea, instant, unsweetened, powder,	72	3%
L	Tea, instant, unsweetened, prepared with water,	0	0%
L	Tea, ready-to-drink, lemon, diet,	0	0%
M	Toaster pastries, brown-sugar-cinnamon,	361	16%
M	Toaster pastries, fruit (includes apple, blueberry, cherry, strawberry),	334	15%
M	Toaster pastries, fruit, frosted (include apples, blueberry, cherry, strawberry),	311	14%
M	Toaster pastries, fruit, toasted (include apple, blueberry, cherry, strawberry),	354	15%
L	Tofu, extra firm, prepared with nigari,	0	0%
L	Tofu, hard, prepared with nigari,	0	0%
V.H	Tofu, salted and fermented (fuyu),	2873	125%
V.H	Tofu, salted and fermented (fuyu), prepared with calcium sulfate,	2873	125%
L	Tomatillos, raw,	0	0%
L	Tomato and vegetable juice, low sodium,	58	3%

M	Tomato juice, canned, with salt added,	253	11%
L	Tomato products, canned, paste, without salt added,	59	3%
M	Tomato products, canned, puree, with salt added,	202	9%
H	Tomato products, canned, sauce,	474	21%
H	Tomato products, canned, sauce, spanish style,	472	21%
H	Tomato products, canned, sauce, with herbs and cheese,	543	24%
M	Tomato products, canned, sauce, with mushrooms,	452	20%
H	Tomato products, canned, sauce, with onions,	551	24%
M	Tomato products, canned, sauce, with onions, green peppers, and celery,	368	16%
M	Tomatoes, crushed, canned,	186	8%
L	Tomatoes, orange, raw,	42	2%
L	Tomatoes, red, ripe, canned, packed in tomato juice,	115	5%
M	Tomatoes, red, ripe, canned, stewed,	221	10%
M	Tomatoes, red, ripe, canned, with green chilies,	401	17%
M	Tomatoes, red, ripe, cooked, stewed,	455	20%
M	Tomatoes, red, ripe, cooked, with salt,	247	11%
L	Tomatoes, red, ripe, raw, year round average,	0	0%
L	Tomatoes, sun-dried,	107	5%
M	Tomatoes, sun-dried, packed in oil, drained,	266	12%
M	Toppings, butterscotch or caramel,	341	15%
L	Toppings, marshmallow cream,	80	3%
L	Toppings, nuts in syrup,	42	2%
L	Toppings, pineapple,	42	2%
M	Tortellini, pasta with cheese filling, fresh-refrigerated, as purchased,	406	18%
H	Tortilla chips, low fat, baked without fat,	517	22%
M	Tortilla chips, yellow, plain, salted,	310	13%
H	Tortilla, blue corn, sakwavikaviki (hopi),	663	29%
H	Tortilla, includes plain and from mutton sandwich (navajo),	482	21%
L	Tortillas, ready-to-bake or -fry, corn,	45	2%

H	Tortillas, ready-to-bake or -fry, flour, refrigerated,	736	32%
H	Tortillas, ready-to-bake or -fry, flour, shelf stable,	742	32%
H	Tortillas, ready-to-bake or -fry, flour, without added calcium,	478	21%
H	Tortillas, ready-to-bake or -fry, whole wheat,	512	22%
H	Tostada shells, corn,	657	29%
M	Tree fern, cooked, with salt,	241	10%
L	Tree fern, cooked, without salt,	0	0%
L	Triticale flour, whole-grain,	0	0%
L	Triticale,	0	0%
H	Turkey and gravy, frozen,	554	24%
H	Turkey breast, low salt, prepackaged or deli, luncheon meat,	772	34%
M	Turkey breast, pre-basted, meat and skin, cooked, roasted,	397	17%
H	Turkey breast, sliced, prepackaged,	922	40%
L	Turkey from whole, dark meat, meat only, raw,	124	5%
L	Turkey from whole, light meat, meat and skin, cooked, roasted,	101	4%
L	Turkey from whole, light meat, meat and skin, raw,	105	5%
M	Turkey from whole, light meat, meat and skin, with added solution, cooked, roasted,	237	10%
M	Turkey from whole, light meat, meat and skin, with added solution, raw,	195	8%
M	Turkey from whole, light meat, meat only, with added solution, cooked, roasted,	238	10%
M	Turkey from whole, light meat, meat only, with added solution, raw,	206	9%
L	Turkey from whole, light meat, raw,	113	5%
M	Turkey from whole, neck, meat only, cooked, simmered,	246	11%
M	Turkey from whole, neck, meat only, raw,	233	10%
M	Turkey pot pie, frozen entree,	350	15%
H	Turkey roast, boneless, frozen, seasoned, light and dark meat, raw,	678	29%
H	Turkey sausage, fresh, cooked,	665	29%

H	Turkey sausage, fresh, raw,	593	26%
H	Turkey sticks, breaded, battered, fried,	838	36%
M	Turkey thigh, pre-basted, meat and skin, cooked, roasted,	437	19%
L	Turkey, all classes, back, meat and skin, cooked, roasted,	73	3%
L	Turkey, all classes, breast, meat and skin, cooked, roasted,	63	3%
L	Turkey, all classes, breast, meat and skin, raw,	59	3%
L	Turkey, all classes, leg, meat and skin, cooked, roasted,	77	3%
L	Turkey, all classes, leg, meat and skin, raw,	74	3%
L	Turkey, all classes, light meat, cooked, roasted,	99	4%
L	Turkey, all classes, wing, meat and skin, cooked, roasted,	61	3%
L	Turkey, all classes, wing, meat and skin, raw,	55	2%
L	Turkey, back from whole bird, meat only, raw,	124	5%
M	Turkey, back, from whole bird, meat and skin, with added solution, raw,	157	7%
M	Turkey, back, from whole bird, meat and skin, with added solution, roasted,	237	10%
L	Turkey, back, from whole bird, meat only, roasted,	104	5%
M	Turkey, back, from whole bird, meat only, with added solution, raw,	167	7%
M	Turkey, back, from whole bird, meat only, with added solution, roasted,	238	10%
L	Turkey, breast, from whole bird, meat only, raw,	113	5%
L	Turkey, breast, from whole bird, meat only, roasted,	99	4%
M	Turkey, breast, from whole bird, meat only, with added solution, raw,	206	9%
M	Turkey, breast, from whole bird, meat only, with added solution, roasted,	238	10%
H	Turkey, breast, smoked, lemon pepper flavor, 97% fat-free,	1160	50%
H	Turkey, canned, meat only, with broth,	518	23%

L	Turkey, dark meat from whole, meat and skin, cooked, roasted,	105	5%
M	Turkey, dark meat from whole, meat and skin, with added solution, cooked, roasted,	206	9%
M	Turkey, dark meat from whole, meat and skin, with added solution, raw,	161	7%
M	Turkey, dark meat from whole, meat only, with added solution, raw,	167	7%
L	Turkey, dark meat, meat and skin, raw,	113	5%
M	Turkey, dark meat, meat only, with added solution, cooked, roasted,	201	9%
H	Turkey, diced, light and dark meat, seasoned,	850	37%
L	Turkey, drumstick, from whole bird, meat only, raw,	113	5%
L	Turkey, drumstick, from whole bird, meat only, roasted,	99	4%
M	Turkey, drumstick, from whole bird, meat only, with added solution, raw,	167	7%
M	Turkey, drumstick, from whole bird, meat only, with added solution, roasted,	201	9%
H	Turkey, drumstick, smoked, cooked, with skin, bone removed,	996	43%
L	Turkey, from whole, dark meat, cooked, roasted,	104	5%
L	Turkey, fryer-roasters, meat and skin, cooked, roasted,	66	3%
M	Turkey, gizzard, all classes, cooked, simmered,	127	6%
M	Turkey, gizzard, all classes, raw,	147	6%
M	Turkey, heart, all classes, cooked, simmered,	140	6%
M	Turkey, heart, all classes, raw,	129	6%
H	Turkey, light or dark meat, smoked, cooked, skin and bone removed,	996	43%
H	Turkey, light or dark meat, smoked, cooked, with skin, bone removed,	996	43%
L	Turkey, liver, all classes, cooked, simmered,	98	4%
M	Turkey, liver, all classes, raw,	131	6%
L	Turkey, mechanically deboned, from turkey frames, raw,	48	2%

L	Turkey, retail parts, breast, meat and skin, cooked, roasted,	114	5%
L	Turkey, retail parts, breast, meat and skin, raw,	72	3%
L	Turkey, retail parts, breast, meat and skin, with added solution, raw,	126	5%
L	Turkey, retail parts, breast, meat only, cooked, roasted,	114	5%
L	Turkey, retail parts, breast, meat only, raw,	74	3%
M	Turkey, retail parts, breast, meat only, with added solution, cooked, roasted,	184	8%
L	Turkey, retail parts, breast, meat only, with added solution, raw,	124	5%
L	Turkey, retail parts, drumstick, meat and skin, cooked, roasted,	112	5%
L	Turkey, retail parts, drumstick, meat and skin, raw,	86	4%
L	Turkey, retail parts, drumstick, meat only, cooked, roasted,	112	5%
L	Turkey, retail parts, drumstick, meat only, raw,	87	4%
L	Turkey, retail parts, thigh, meat and skin, cooked, roasted,	101	4%
L	Turkey, retail parts, thigh, meat and skin, raw,	75	3%
L	Turkey, retail parts, thigh, meat only, cooked, roasted,	104	5%
L	Turkey, retail parts, thigh, meat only, raw,	75	3%
L	Turkey, retail parts, wing, meat and skin, cooked, roasted,	106	5%
L	Turkey, retail parts, wing, meat and skin, raw,	67	3%
L	Turkey, retail parts, wing, meat only, cooked, roasted,	103	4%
L	Turkey, retail parts, wing, meat only, raw,	69	3%
L	Turkey, skin from whole (light and dark), roasted,	116	5%
M	Turkey, skin from whole (light and dark), with added solution, raw,	138	6%
L	Turkey, skin from whole, (light and dark), raw,	62	3%
M	Turkey, skin from whole, (light and dark), with added solution, roasted,	234	10%

L	Turkey, skin, from retail parts, from dark meat, cooked, roasted,	106	5%
L	Turkey, skin, from retail parts, from dark meat, raw,	78	3%
M	Turkey, stuffing, mashed potatoes w\gravy, assorted vegetables, frozen, microwaved,	326	14%
L	Turkey, thigh, from whole bird, meat only, raw,	124	5%
L	Turkey, thigh, from whole bird, meat only, roasted,	104	5%
M	Turkey, thigh, from whole bird, meat only, with added solution, raw,	167	7%
M	Turkey, thigh, from whole bird, meat only, with added solution, roasted,	201	9%
H	Turkey, white, rotisserie, deli cut,	1200	52%
L	Turkey, whole, giblets, cooked, simmered,	117	5%
M	Turkey, whole, giblets, raw,	136	6%
L	Turkey, whole, meat and skin, cooked, roasted,	103	4%
L	Turkey, whole, meat and skin, raw,	112	5%
M	Turkey, whole, meat and skin, with added solution, raw,	180	8%
M	Turkey, whole, meat and skin, with added solution, roasted,	224	10%
L	Turkey, whole, meat only, cooked, roasted,	101	4%
L	Turkey, whole, meat only, raw,	118	5%
M	Turkey, whole, meat only, with added solution, raw,	194	8%
M	Turkey, whole, meat only, with added solution, roasted,	223	10%
L	Turkey, wing, from whole bird, meat only, raw,	113	5%
L	Turkey, wing, from whole bird, meat only, roasted,	99	4%
M	Turkey, wing, from whole bird, meat only, with added solution, raw,	206	9%
M	Turkey, wing, from whole bird, meat only, with added solution, roasted,	238	10%
H	Turkey, wing, smoked, cooked, with skin, bone removed,	996	43%

L	Turkey, young hen, skin only, cooked, roasted,	44	2%
M	Turnip greens and turnips, frozen, cooked, boiled, drained, with salt,	255	11%
M	Turnip greens, canned, solids and liquids,	277	12%
M	Turnip greens, cooked, boiled, drained, with salt,	265	12%
M	Turnip greens, frozen, cooked, boiled, drained, with salt,	251	11%
L	Turnip greens, raw,	40	2%
M	Turnips, cooked, boiled, drained, with salt,	286	12%
M	Turnips, frozen, cooked, boiled, drained, with salt,	272	12%
L	Turnips, frozen, cooked, boiled, drained, without salt,	36	2%
L	Turnips, raw,	67	3%
H	Turnover, cheese-filled, tomato-based sauce, frozen, unprepared,	598	26%
M	Turnover, chicken- or turkey-, and vegetable-filled, reduced fat, frozen,	276	12%
M	Turnover, filled with egg, meat and cheese, frozen,	378	16%
M	Turnover, meat- and cheese-filled, tomato-based sauce, reduced fat, frozen,	378	16%
L	Turtle, green, raw,	68	3%
L	Vanilla extract, imitation, alcohol,	0	0%
L	Vanilla extract, imitation, no alcohol,	0	0%
L	Veal, australian, rib, rib roast, separable lean and fat, raw,	76	3%
L	Veal, australian, rib, rib roast, separable lean only, raw,	83	4%
L	Veal, australian, separable fat, raw,	44	2%
L	Veal, australian, shank, fore, bone-in, separable lean and fat, raw,	108	5%
L	Veal, australian, shank, fore, bone-in, separable lean only, raw,	112	5%
L	Veal, australian, shank, hind, bone-in, separable lean and fat,	95	4%
L	Veal, australian, shank, hind, bone-in, separable lean only, raw,	98	4%

L	Veal, breast, plate half, boneless, separable lean and fat, cooked, braised,	64	3%
L	Veal, breast, point half, boneless, separable lean and fat, cooked, braised,	66	3%
L	Veal, breast, separable fat, cooked,	49	2%
L	Veal, breast, whole, boneless, separable lean and fat, cooked, braised,	65	3%
L	Veal, breast, whole, boneless, separable lean and fat, raw,	71	3%
L	Veal, breast, whole, boneless, separable lean only, cooked, braised,	68	3%
L	Veal, composite of trimmed retail cuts, separable fat, cooked,	57	2%
L	Veal, composite of trimmed retail cuts, separable lean and fat, cooked,	87	4%
L	Veal, composite of trimmed retail cuts, separable lean and fat, raw,	82	4%
L	Veal, composite of trimmed retail cuts, separable lean only, cooked,	89	4%
L	Veal, composite of trimmed retail cuts, separable lean only, raw,	86	4%
L	Veal, cubed for stew (leg and shoulder), separable lean only, cooked, braised,	93	4%
L	Veal, cubed for stew (leg and shoulder), separable lean only, raw,	83	4%
L	Veal, foreshank, osso buco, separable lean and fat, cooked, braised,	90	4%
L	Veal, foreshank, osso buco, separable lean only, cooked, braised,	90	4%
L	Veal, ground, cooked, broiled,	83	4%
M	Veal, ground, cooked, pan-fried,	146	6%
L	Veal, ground, raw,	103	4%
L	Veal, leg (top round), separable lean and fat, cooked, braised,	67	3%
M	Veal, leg (top round), separable lean and fat, cooked, pan-fried, breaded,	454	20%
L	Veal, leg (top round), separable lean and fat, cooked, pan-fried, not breaded,	76	3%
L	Veal, leg (top round), separable lean and fat, cooked, roasted,	68	3%

L	Veal, leg (top round), separable lean and fat, raw,	63	3%
L	Veal, leg (top round), separable lean only, cooked, braised,	67	3%
M	Veal, leg (top round), separable lean only, cooked, pan-fried, breaded,	455	20%
L	Veal, leg (top round), separable lean only, cooked, pan-fried, not breaded,	77	3%
L	Veal, leg (top round), separable lean only, cooked, roasted,	68	3%
L	Veal, leg (top round), separable lean only, raw,	64	3%
L	Veal, leg, top round, cap off, cutlet, boneless, cooked, grilled,	88	4%
L	Veal, leg, top round, cap off, cutlet, boneless, raw,	86	4%
L	Veal, loin, chop, separable lean and fat, cooked, grilled,	86	4%
L	Veal, loin, chop, separable lean only, cooked, grilled,	85	4%
L	Veal, loin, separable lean and fat, cooked, braised,	80	3%
L	Veal, loin, separable lean and fat, cooked, roasted,	93	4%
L	Veal, loin, separable lean and fat, raw,	98	4%
L	Veal, loin, separable lean only, cooked, braised,	84	4%
L	Veal, loin, separable lean only, cooked, roasted,	96	4%
L	Veal, loin, separable lean only, raw,	99	4%
L	Veal, rib, separable lean and fat, cooked, braised,	95	4%
L	Veal, rib, separable lean and fat, cooked, roasted,	92	4%
L	Veal, rib, separable lean and fat, raw,	89	4%
L	Veal, rib, separable lean only, cooked, braised,	99	4%
L	Veal, rib, separable lean only, cooked, roasted,	97	4%
L	Veal, rib, separable lean only, raw,	95	4%

L	Veal, shank (fore and hind), separable lean and fat, cooked, braised,	93	4%
L	Veal, shank (fore and hind), separable lean and fat, raw,	84	4%
L	Veal, shank (fore and hind), separable lean only, cooked, braised,	94	4%
L	Veal, shank (fore and hind), separable lean only, raw,	85	4%
L	Veal, shank, separable lean and fat, raw,	107	5%
L	Veal, shank, separable lean only, raw,	109	5%
L	Veal, shoulder, arm, separable lean and fat, cooked, braised,	87	4%
L	Veal, shoulder, arm, separable lean and fat, cooked, roasted,	90	4%
L	Veal, shoulder, arm, separable lean and fat, raw,	83	4%
L	Veal, shoulder, arm, separable lean only, cooked, braised,	90	4%
L	Veal, shoulder, arm, separable lean only, cooked, roasted,	91	4%
L	Veal, shoulder, arm, separable lean only, raw,	86	4%
L	Veal, shoulder, blade chop, separable lean and fat, cooked, grilled,	111	5%
L	Veal, shoulder, blade chop, separable lean and fat, raw,	91	4%
L	Veal, shoulder, blade chop, separable lean only, cooked, grilled,	113	5%
L	Veal, shoulder, blade chop, separable lean only, raw,	92	4%
L	Veal, shoulder, blade, separable lean and fat, cooked, braised,	98	4%
L	Veal, shoulder, blade, separable lean and fat, cooked, roasted,	100	4%
L	Veal, shoulder, blade, separable lean only, cooked, braised,	101	4%
L	Veal, shoulder, blade, separable lean only, cooked, roasted,	102	4%
L	Veal, shoulder, whole (arm and blade), separable lean and fat, cooked, braised,	95	4%

L	Veal, shoulder, whole (arm and blade), separable lean and fat, cooked, roasted,	96	4%
L	Veal, shoulder, whole (arm and blade), separable lean and fat, raw,	91	4%
L	Veal, shoulder, whole (arm and blade), separable lean only, cooked, braised,	97	4%
L	Veal, shoulder, whole (arm and blade), separable lean only, cooked, roasted,	97	4%
L	Veal, shoulder, whole (arm and blade), separable lean only, raw,	92	4%
L	Veal, sirloin, separable lean and fat, cooked, braised,	79	3%
L	Veal, sirloin, separable lean and fat, cooked, roasted,	83	4%
L	Veal, sirloin, separable lean and fat, raw,	76	3%
L	Veal, sirloin, separable lean only, cooked, braised,	81	4%
L	Veal, sirloin, separable lean only, cooked, roasted,	85	4%
L	Veal, sirloin, separable lean only, raw,	80	3%
M	Veal, variety meats and by-products, brain, cooked, braised,	156	7%
M	Veal, variety meats and by-products, brain, cooked, pan-fried,	176	8%
M	Veal, variety meats and by-products, brain, raw,	127	6%
L	Veal, variety meats and by-products, heart, cooked, braised,	58	3%
L	Veal, variety meats and by-products, heart, raw,	77	3%
L	Veal, variety meats and by-products, kidneys, cooked, braised,	110	5%
M	Veal, variety meats and by-products, kidneys, raw,	178	8%
L	Veal, variety meats and by-products, liver, cooked, braised,	78	3%
L	Veal, variety meats and by-products, liver, cooked, pan-fried,	85	4%
L	Veal, variety meats and by-products, liver, raw,	77	3%

L	Veal, variety meats and by-products, lungs, cooked, braised,	56	2%
L	Veal, variety meats and by-products, lungs, raw,	108	5%
L	Veal, variety meats and by-products, pancreas, cooked, braised,	68	3%
L	Veal, variety meats and by-products, pancreas, raw,	67	3%
L	Veal, variety meats and by-products, spleen, cooked, braised,	58	3%
L	Veal, variety meats and by-products, spleen, raw,	97	4%
L	Veal, variety meats and by-products, thymus, cooked, braised,	59	3%
L	Veal, variety meats and by-products, thymus, raw,	67	3%
L	Veal, variety meats and by-products, tongue, cooked, braised,	64	3%
L	Veal, variety meats and by-products, tongue, raw,	82	4%
M	Vegetable juice cocktail, canned,	169	7%
L	Vegetable juice cocktail, low sodium, canned,	55	2%
H	Vegetable oil-butter spread, reduced calorie,	581	25%
L	Vegetable oil, palm kernel,	0	0%
M	Vegetables, mixed, canned, drained solids,	214	9%
M	Vegetables, mixed, canned, solids and liquids,	224	10%
M	Vegetables, mixed, frozen, cooked, boiled, drained, with salt,	271	12%
L	Vegetables, mixed, frozen, unprepared,	47	2%
H	Vegetarian fillets,	490	21%
H	Vegetarian meatloaf or patties,	550	24%
H	Veggie burgers or soyburgers, unprepared,	569	25%
L	Vermicelli, made from soy,	0	0%
L	Vinegar, cider,	0	0%
L	Vinegar, distilled,	0	0%
L	Vitasoy usa nasoya, lite silken tofu,	79	3%
L	Vitasoy usa, vitasoy light vanilla soymilk,	49	2%
L	Vitasoy usa, vitasoy organic classic original soymilk,	66	3%

L	Vitasoy usa, vitasoy organic creamy original soymilk,	66	3%
H	Waffle, buttermilk, frozen, ready-to-heat, microwaved,	663	29%
H	Waffle, buttermilk, frozen, ready-to-heat, toasted,	710	31%
H	Waffle, plain, frozen, ready-to-heat, microwave,	682	30%
H	Waffles, buttermilk, frozen, ready-to-heat,	621	27%
H	Waffles, chocolate chip, frozen, ready-to-heat,	529	23%
H	Waffles, gluten-free, frozen, ready-to-heat,	505	22%
H	Waffles, plain, frozen, ready -to-heat, toasted,	730	32%
H	Waffles, plain, frozen, ready-to-heat,	638	28%
H	Waffles, plain, prepared from recipe,	511	22%
H	Waffles, whole wheat, lowfat, frozen, ready-to-heat,	557	24%
V.H	Wasabi,	3390	147%
L	Water, bottled, generic,	0	0%
L	Water, tap, drinking,	0	0%
L	Water, tap, municipal,	0	0%
L	Water, tap, well,	0	0%
L	Watercress, raw,	41	2%
L	Watermelon, raw,	0	0%
M	Waxgourd, (chinese preserving melon), cooked, boiled, drained, with salt,	343	15%
L	Waxgourd, (chinese preserving melon), cooked, boiled, drained, without salt,	107	5%
L	Waxgourd, (chinese preserving melon), raw,	111	5%
M	Whale, beluga, meat, dried (alaska native),	220	10%
L	Wheat bran, crude,	0	0%
L	Wheat flour, white, all-purpose, enriched, bleached,	0	0%
L	Wheat flour, white, all-purpose, enriched, calcium-fortified,	0	0%
L	Wheat flour, white, all-purpose, enriched, unbleached,	0	0%
H	Wheat flour, white, all-purpose, self-rising, enriched,	1193	52%
L	Wheat flour, white, all-purpose, unenriched,	0	0%

L	Wheat flour, white, bread, enriched,	0	0%
L	Wheat flour, white, cake, enriched,	0	0%
H	Wheat flour, white, tortilla mix, enriched,	677	29%
L	Wheat flour, whole-grain,	0	0%
L	Wheat flours, bread, unenriched,	0	0%
L	Wheat, durum,	0	0%
L	Wheat, hard red spring,	0	0%
L	Wheat, hard red winter,	0	0%
L	Wheat, hard white,	0	0%
L	Wheat, soft red winter,	0	0%
L	Wheat, soft white,	0	0%
M	Whey protein powder isolate,	372	16%
H	Whey, acid, dried,	968	42%
L	Whey, acid, fluid,	48	2%
H	Whey, sweet, dried,	1079	47%
L	Whey, sweet, fluid,	54	2%
L	Whipped cream substitute, dietetic, made from powdered mix,	106	5%
L	Whipped topping, frozen, low fat,	72	3%
L	Whiskey sour mix, bottled,	102	4%
M	Whiskey sour mix, powder,	274	12%
L	Wild rice, cooked,	0	0%
M	Winged bean, immature seeds, cooked, boiled, drained, with salt,	240	10%
L	Winged beans, immature seeds, cooked, boiled, drained, without salt,	0	0%
L	Winged beans, immature seeds, raw,	0	0%
M	Winged beans, mature seeds, cooked, boiled, with salt,	249	11%
L	Winged beans, mature seeds, raw,	38	2%
H	Wonton wrappers (includes egg roll wrappers),	572	25%
H	Yachtwurst, with pistachio nuts, cooked,	936	41%
M	Yam, cooked, boiled, drained, or baked, with salt,	244	11%
L	Yambean (jicama), raw,	0	0%
M	Yardlong bean, cooked, boiled, drained, with salt,	240	10%
L	Yardlong bean, cooked, boiled, drained, without salt,	0	0%

L	Yardlong bean, raw,	0	0%
M	Yardlong beans, mature seeds, cooked, boiled, with salt,	241	10%
L	Yardlong beans, mature seeds, cooked, boiled, without salt,	0	0%
V.H	Yeast extract spread,	3380	147%
H	Yellow rice with seasoning, dry packet mix, unprepared,	1316	57%
L	Yogurt parfait, lowfat, with fruit and granola,	49	2%
M	Yogurt, chocolate, nonfat milk,	135	6%
M	Yogurt, chocolate, nonfat milk, fortified with vitamin d,	135	6%
L	Yogurt, frozen, flavors not chocolate, nonfat milk, with low-calorie sweetener,	81	4%
L	Yogurt, fruit variety, nonfat,	58	3%
L	Yogurt, fruit variety, nonfat, fortified with vitamin d,	58	3%
L	Yogurt, fruit, low fat, 10 grams protein per. 8 ounce,	58	3%
L	Yogurt, fruit, low fat, 10 grams protein per 8 ounce, fortified with vitamin d,	58	3%
L	Yogurt, fruit, low fat, 11 grams protein per 8 ounce,	65	3%
L	Yogurt, fruit, low fat, 9 grams protein per 8 ounce,	53	2%
L	Yogurt, fruit, low fat, 9 grams protein per 8 ounce, fortified with vitamin d,	53	2%
L	Yogurt, fruit, lowfat, with low calorie sweetener,	58	3%
L	Yogurt, fruit, lowfat, with low calorie sweetener, fortified with vitamin d,	58	3%
L	Yogurt, greek, plain, nonfat,	36	2%
L	Yogurt, plain, low fat, 12 grams protein per 8 ounce,	70	3%
L	Yogurt, plain, skim milk, 13 grams protein per 8 ounce,	77	3%
L	Yogurt, plain, whole milk, 8 grams protein per 8 ounce,	46	2%
L	Yogurt, vanilla flavor, lowfat milk, sweetened with low calorie sweetener,	66	3%

L	Yogurt, vanilla or lemon flavor, nonfat milk, sweetened with low-calorie sweetener,	59	3%
L	Yogurt, vanilla or lemon flavor, nonfat milk, sweetened with low-calorie sweetener, fortified with vitamin d,	59	3%
L	Yogurt, vanilla, low fat, 11 grams protein per 8 ounce,	66	3%
L	Yogurt, vanilla, low fat, 11 grams protein per 8 ounce, fortified with vitamin d,	66	3%
L	Yogurt, vanilla, non-fat,	47	2%
L	Yokan, prepared from adzuki beans and sugar,	83	4%
L	Zucchini, baby, raw,	0	0%
M	Zucchini, includes skin, cooked, boiled, drained, with salt,	239	10%
L	Zucchini, includes skin, cooked, boiled, drained, without salt,	0	0%
M	Zucchini, includes skin, frozen, cooked, boiled, drained, with salt,	238	10%
L	Zucchini, includes skin, frozen, cooked, boiled, drained, without salt,	0	0%
L	Zucchini, includes skin, frozen, unprepared,	0	0%
M	Zucchini, italian style, canned,	374	16%
M	Zwieback,	227	10%

Made in the USA
Columbia, SC
27 March 2022

58221968R00085